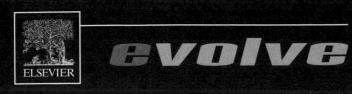

:• *To access your Student Resources, visit:*

http://evolve.elsevier.com/Daniel

Evolve Student Learning Resources for *Daniel: Mosby's Dental Hygiene: Concepts, Cases, and Competencies, Second Edition* offers the following features:

Student Resources

- **Patient Education handouts** - Customizable handouts you can print and take with you to clinic

- **Clinical resource tables** - Organized information on state licensure boards, dentifrices, and more—up-to-date and at your fingertips!

- **Comprehensive health history form** - Now use this standard form from the text to practice recording patient information!

- **Patient record forms** - Forms from the Companion CD-ROM patients are available for extra review!

- **Suggested agencies and websites** - Internet resource links for further learning

- **Additional readings and resources** - Extended chapter-by-chapter bibliographies useful in research and study

- **Competencies for Entry into the Profession of Dental Hygiene as approved by the 2003 House of Delegates**

Clinical Companion Study Guide For

Mosby's Dental Hygiene: Concepts, Cases, and Competencies

Second Edition

Bonnie Francis, RDH, MS
Adjunct Clinical Associate Professor
Department of Dental Ecology
University of North Carolina
School of Dentistry
Chapel Hill, North Carolina
Dallas, Texas

Shannon H. Mitchell, RDH, MS
Adjunct Clinical Associate Professor
University of North Carolina
School of Dentistry
Chapel Hill, North Carolina

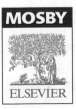

MOSBY

ELSEVIER

MOSBY
ELSEVIER

11830 Westline Industrial Drive
St. Louis, Missouri 63146

CLINICAL COMPANION STUDY GUIDE FOR MOSBY'S
DENTAL HYGIENE: CONCEPTS, CASES,
AND COMPETENCIES
(by: Susan J. Daniel, Sherry A. Harfst, Rebecca S. Wilder)   ISBN: 978-0-323-04534-6
Copyright © 2008, 2004 by Mosby, Inc., an affiliate of Elsevier Inc.

ISBN-13: 978-0-323-04534-6
ISBN-10: 0-323-04534-0

Vice President and Publisher: Linda Duncan
Senior Editor: John Dolan
Developmental Editor: Julie Nebel
Publishing Services Manager: Julie Eddy
Project Manager: Laura Loveall
Cover Art: Margaret Reid

Printed in United States of America

Last digit is the print number: 9 8 7 6 5 4 3 2 1

Contents

Introduction

Mosby's Dental Hygiene: Concepts, Cases, and Competencies provides a unique approach to the educational process of the dental hygienist. This comprehensive package offers faculty and students a learning environment in a textbook, CD-ROM, *Clinical Companion Study Guide,* and Evolve web site that support case-based and competency-based education. (See the Preface in the textbook for more details about each of these components.) This *Clinical Companion Study Guide* is a resource that incorporates many creative features within the package elements to enhance each student's education.

Every chapter in this manual is organized in a consistent manner to clarify the learning process. While studying the text, students can explore the other resources at their individual paces, using this clinical companion as a guide. All pages are perforated; therefore completed worksheets and other helpful information can be laminated and taken into clinical practice or included as part of a student portfolio.

A full listing of the additional materials found on Evolve is located on the first page of this publication—extra copies of Critical Thinking Activity worksheets and full-size Process Performance Forms are only the beginning. It is our hope that all students will benefit from using the resources contained in this package, allowing students to integrate their knowledge into clinical practice. In addition, we hope this resource will truly be a clinical companion as students begin their careers in dental hygiene.

—Bonnie Francis
—Shannon H. Mitchell

1 The Dental Hygiene Profession

WHY do I need to know about The Dental Hygiene Profession?

Study of the history of the dental profession provides a window into the past that helps clarify the present. The history of the development of the dental hygiene profession has always emphasized prevention of disease and promotion of health. This rich heritage sets the stage for the profession's contributions as preventive dental care specialists.

WHAT will I be able to do with this knowledge?

1. Appreciate the value of the history of the dental hygiene profession.
2. Understand the process necessary to become a licensed professional.
3. Develop educational goals for the first term of dental hygiene.
4. Create a student portfolio.
5. Develop an appreciation for the profession of dental hygiene and professional associations.

HOW do I prepare myself to transfer this knowledge to patient care?

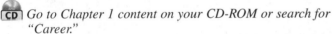 *Go to Chapter 1 content on your CD-ROM or search for "Career."*

These CD-ROM exercises support the concepts presented in this chapter, five of which are actually written to your student Portfolio. The exercises take the concepts of professionalism to a personal level. You are asked to explore career path options and are connected via web addresses with dental hygiene programs around the country. Through these exercises, you are introduced to the Portfolio feature as a professional development tool. Based on licensing parameters for your (or a given) state, research and record information pertaining to continuing education, dental hygiene organizations, and licensed duties. Once recorded, this information can be stored in your student Portfolio.

CD Exercises

■ *1-1: Career Mobility and Career Choices: Meet the Authors:* Read short statements from the authors about their overview of the profession.
■ *1-2: Career Mobility and Career Choices—Video:* Explore all the career paths open to dental hygiene

professionals, review each path, and present an individual view of this role.

Portfolio Features

■ *1-A: Types of Degrees:* Explore Internet listings of dental education programs in the United States and Canada.
■ *1-B: Licensure and Regulations:* Record and assess legal functions within the scope of your state practice act.
■ *1-C: Continuing Education:* Determine and record the continuing dental education requirements for licensure in your state.
■ *1-D: Professional Organizations:* Research and archive national and local associations for future networking.
■ *1-E: Student Portfolio:* Provides an overview of portfolio concept, entering primary information.
■ *1-F: Student Portfolio: Health Belief Checklist, Personal Health History, Personal Prevention Survey:* Complete a personal assessment of your current perception of health; document your current health status—to be reviewed periodically; document your current dental health, fluoride survey, diet survey, beliefs, and behaviors.

Textbook

Review Case Study 1-1, Advances in Dental Technology, and the case applications.

HOW do I perform these skills?

evolve

A printable version of this checklist is available on your Evolve Student Resources.

To understand and value the dental hygiene profession successfully, I will:

☐ Identify the number, locations, and degrees offered in dental education programs in the United States and Canada.

☐ Describe the legal functions within the scope of my state practice act.

☐ Evaluate all career paths open to dental hygiene professionals.

☐ Determine and record the continuing dental education requirements for licensure in my state.

☐ Research and archive national and local associations for future networking.

☐ Use the Internet as a source for information and links to search engines, for example, PubMed and dentally focused web sites, to perform literature reviews.

HOW can I more effectively use this knowledge?

Critical Thinking Activities

Use the following worksheets to complete activities #1 and #3.

1. Using Worksheet #1, ask your faculty, colleagues, dentist, dental hygienist, or the dental hygiene association to identify a local dental hygienist that has been in practice for longer than 20 years. Call and introduce yourself, and ask for an interview on the topic of dental hygiene—then and now. Determine the nature of the changes the dental hygienist has witnessed in the following areas: sterilization, staffing, staff interaction, uniforms, equipment, use of technology, emphasis in practice, educational requirements, and licensing process.

    Which areas have seen the most change?

    Which areas have seen the least change?

    Compare your findings with those of a classmate who has interviewed a different hygienist with a similar career history.

2. Review the concept of the dental hygiene portfolio discussed in this chapter. Make a list of potential portfolio folders from your most recent educational accomplishments. Would such a portfolio have been helpful to your interview process on entering the dental hygiene program?

3. Using Worksheet #2, observe dental hygienists in different work settings such as those listed below. List the advantages and disadvantages of that role.
    Clinician
    Administrator or manager
    Educator
    Researcher
    Advocate
    Public health

4. Are you interested in pursuing a career in areas other than clinical dental hygiene? Do you think a mentor—someone already accomplished in that area of dental hygiene practice—would be helpful to you? If yes, how do you see that relationship starting?

5. Determine your state's continuing education (CE) requirements. Which CE courses are offered at your school? Is a college or university within driving distance at which you could attend a course? Does your school require you to keep track of any CE courses you take? Do you see any benefit tracking CE courses as a student?

6. If your school has provided you with competency statements that are specific to your program, which of those competencies does Chapter 1 address?

Worksheet #1

Record your findings from Critical Thinking Activity #1 on this interview form. In the columns to the right, indicate which areas have seen the most change and the least change in the columns provided.

Note the Changes Reported in the Following Areas	Most Changed	Least Changed
Sterilization	☐	☐
Staffing	☐	☐
Staff interaction	☐	☐
Uniforms	☐	☐
Equipment	☐	☐
Use of technology	☐	☐
Emphasis in practice	☐	☐
Educational requirements	☐	☐
Licensing process	☐	☐

Dental hygienist's name: _____ Year of graduation: _____

Certificate or degree received from: _____

Additional notes and observations:

_____

_____

_____

_____

_____

_____

_____

_____

_____

_____

3

Worksheet #2

Looking at Critical Thinking Activity #3, list the different roles and what you personally believe to be their advantages and disadvantages.

Roles	Advantages	Disadvantages
Clinician		
Administrator or manager		
Educator		
Researcher		
Advocate		
Public health		

DO I have all the answers?

Review Questions

Check your answers against the Answer Key at the back of this Study Guide to assess what you have learned.

1. All of the following components of dentistry have changed dramatically since the 1900s *except* for which one?
   a. Professional attire
   b. Patient and operator positioning
   c. Equipment
   d. Need for better communication

2. Which one of the following individuals is credited with being the founder of dental hygiene?
   a. Irene Newman
   b. Alfred Fones
   c. D.D. Smith
   d. Robin Adair

3. In which of the following areas of dentistry are most dental hygienists employed?
   a. Periodontal practices
   b. General dental practices
   c. Public health dentistry
   d. Pediatric dentistry

4. Dental hygienists practice their career under all *except* which one of the following levels of supervision?
   a. Independent
   b. Direct
   c. Modified direct
   d. General

5. Oral and systemic health are related by which of the following mechanisms?
   a. Immune components
   b. Treatments
   c. Prevention strategies
   d. Diseases

6. Dental hygiene programs can be found in which one of the following institutions?
   a. Universities
   b. Community colleges
   c. Technical institutes
   d. All of the above

7. The process for developing competence while in a dental hygiene education program can be measured by which one of the following?
   a. Faculty mentor
   b. Goals
   c. Competencies
   d. Documentation of performance
   e. All of the above

8. Changes in licensure and supervision of dental hygienists are primarily driven by which one of the following reasons?
   a. Access to care issues
   b. Need for larger quantity of dental hygienists
   c. Dental hygienists request the changes
   d. Dental boards want the changes

WHERE do I go for more information or support?

evolve

For suggested web sites and agencies, additional readings and resources, and more chapter-specific information, please consult your Evolve Student Resources. Because of the ever-changing nature of the Internet, please keep in mind that web sites listed and their content may change.

CD-ROM

Reference files: As you work through the CD-ROM exercises, you should be able to print reference files and add them to your class materials. No specific reference files apply to this chapter.

HOW can I keep track of my progress toward competence?

As an ongoing picture of progress, record and monitor clinical experiences relating to Chapter 1 content in your Portfolio.

Self-Reflection

On a regular basis, review these experiences (with a faculty member). Identify strengths, weaknesses (not just numbers related to clinical requirements), and changes that you would incorporate into your clinical care plan now that you have had these experiences.

2 Health Promotion: A Basis of Practice

WHY do I need to know about Health Promotion: A Basis of Practice?

The dental hygienist's role in health care is exemplified as one who can promote health through prevention and intervention. Possessing knowledge of health theory, health behavior, and the mechanism for change is key to health promotion in the dental hygiene practice. This chapter provides dental hygienists with the foundation for their roles as the promoters of appropriate healthcare habits and behaviors for patients.

WHAT will I be able to do with this knowledge?

1. Determine working definitions for *health* and *health promotion*.
2. Discuss the paradigm shift with regard to health promotion in dental hygiene.
3. Apply theoretical models of health behavior to plan interventions aimed at changing health behaviors.
4. State general demographic parameters of an epidemiologic survey.
5. Describe the burden of oral disease in the U.S. population.
6. Discuss the two national health planning reports and their implications for dental hygienists for improving both individual and population health.

HOW do I prepare myself to transfer this knowledge to patient care?

Textbook

Review Case Study 2-1, Expanding the Definition of Health, and the case applications.

For important concepts and application of knowledge, Box 2-6 and Figures 2-2 through 2-13 may be especially helpful for clinical transfer and may be used as a clinical resource.

HOW do I perform these skills?

evolve

A printable version of this checklist is available on your Evolve Student Resources.

To communicate health promotion during patient care successfully, I will:

- ☐ Review the oral risk assessment prevention survey.
- ☐ Review intraoral findings.
- ☐ Clearly identify risk factors that place an individual at risk for developing oral or systemic diseases.
- ☐ Discuss risk factors with the patient.
- ☐ Communicate preventive measures to the patient.
- ☐ Discuss health practices that can help the patient attain a higher quality of life.
- ☐ Document findings and procedure in chart.

HOW can I more effectively use this knowledge?

Critical Thinking Activities

Use the following worksheet to complete activity #2.

1. With a study partner, review the medical histories of several clinic patients. Select several health promotion topics, and present your conclusions to a faculty member and fellow student. Describe their feedback.
2. Using Worksheet #1, develop a personal philosophy of practice. Include such topics as services you will provide, processes you will use to determine the best approach to health promotion for your patients, and the exact ways you plan to promote health. Place your personal philosophy of practice into your portfolio.
3. "You have the ability to touch a life." In the context of this chapter, what is the meaning of this phrase?
4. Oral health is related to well-being and the quality of life as measured by functional, psychosocial, and economic dimensions. What does this statement mean to the clinical practice of dental hygiene?
5. Survey 10 classmates. Ask whether in the last 6 months they have experienced orofacial pain in any of the following categories:
   Toothache
   Oral sores
   Jaw joint
   Face and cheek
   Burning mouth
   How consistent are your findings with the statistical prevalence of these conditions as reported in the text?
6. With a group of four classmates, select one of the goals from *Healthy People 2010* and one of the action steps from the Surgeon General's report. Develop an action plan for your class, based on a community-level health theory. Explain how you would execute your strategies.

Worksheet #1

Use this worksheet with Critical Thinking Activity #2. Also include your definition of health.

Statement of Philosophy

Goal statement: As a licensed dental professional, I will (how you plan to function in the oral health care environment, relationships with employer or employers, co-workers, patients):

_____

_____

_____

_____

Services I will provide:

_____

_____

_____

_____

Processes I will use to determine the effectiveness of my approach to health promotion:

_____

_____

_____

_____

Ways in which I plan to promote health:

_____

_____

_____

_____

My definition of health:

_____

_____

_____

_____

Chapter **2** **Health Promotion: A Basis of Practice**

DO I have all the answers?

Review Questions

Check your answers against the Answer Key at the back of this Study Guide to assess what you have learned.

1. Significant progress in the reduction of the incidence, prevalence, and severity of dental caries has been the result of which one of the following community-based programs?
   a. Community water fluoridation
   b. Dental sealants
   c. School-based topical fluoride programs
   d. *a* and *b*
   e. All of the above
2. Health is best defined as which one of the following?
   a. Quality of life
   b. Absence of disease
   c. Complete state of physical, mental, and social well-being
   d. All of the above
3. Which one of the following individual health theories attempts to explain the relationship between attitudes and behaviors?
   a. Health Belief Model (HBM)
   b. Diffusion of Innovation Theory (DIT)
   c. Theory of Reasoned Action (TRA)
   d. Social Cognitive Theory (SCT)
   e. All of the above
4. Knowledge is the single-most important determinant for changing health behaviors.
   a. True
   b. False
5. The most recent national health survey (National Health and Nutrition Examination Survey [NHANES] III, 1988-1994) validates which one of the following statements?
   a. Dental caries is five times more common than asthma.
   b. Dental caries is equally evident across all socio-economic guidelines.
   c. Dental caries represents the single-most chronic childhood disease.
   d. *a* and *c*
   e. All of the above

6. Which one of the following statements is/are *true?*
   a. The mouth reflects the general health and well-being of an individual.
   b. Oral diseases and conditions are associated with general health problems.
   c. Despite improvements in oral health status, profound disparities still exist in some population groups.
   d. Many systemic diseases and conditions have oral manifestations.
   e. All of the above

WHERE do I go for more information or support?

evolve

For suggested web sites and agencies, additional readings and resources, and more chapter-specific information, please consult your Evolve Student Resources. Because of the ever-changing nature of the Internet, please keep in mind that web sites listed and their content may change.

CD-ROM

Reference files: As you work through the CD-ROM exercises, you should be able to print reference files and add them to your class materials. No specific reference files apply to this chapter.

HOW can I keep track of my progress toward competence?

As an ongoing picture of progress, record and monitor clinical experiences relating to Chapter 2 content in your Portfolio.

Self-Reflection

On a regular basis, review these experiences (with a faculty member). Identify strengths, weaknesses (not just numbers), and changes that you would incorporate into your clinical care plan now that you have had these experiences.

3 Legal and Ethical Considerations

WHY do I need to know about Legal and Ethical Considerations?

Society places trust in health professionals, and with that trust comes a set of expectations that the professional will work for the good of the public he or she serves. Some of these expectations are codified into laws and regulations, and some are spelled out in professional standards of conduct. As with other health professionals, the conduct of a dental hygienist is bound by legal statutes, regulations, and ethical guidelines.

WHAT will I be able to do with this knowledge?

1. Discuss the ethical principles that guide dental hygiene practice.
2. Define *informed consent*, explaining why it is important to the patient and the dental healthcare provider.
3. Identify the elements a plaintiff must prove in a lawsuit based on tort law.
4. Define *battery*.
5. Describe how the First Amendment to the U.S. Constitution may relate to the medical care an individual receives.
6. State the steps that must be taken in the termination of a patient from care to protect the healthcare provider from charges of abandonment.
7. Understand the value of *medical directives*, and describe their purpose in health care.
8. Explain the application of *risk management* in dental hygiene care.
9. List possible legal risks in the practice of dental hygiene.
10. Document the dental hygiene process of care with regard to informed consent.
11. Apply the concept *standard of care* to dental hygiene patient care.
12. Discuss the role of the regulatory agency in dental hygiene practice.

HOW do I prepare myself to transfer this knowledge to patient care?

 Go to Chapter 3 content on your CD-ROM or search for "Legal."

CD Exercises
Determine whether each principle or value presented has been breached or upheld in the following exercises:
- *3-1: Ethical Principles in Dental Hygiene—Ann Cronin*
- *3-2: Ethical Principles in Dental Hygiene—George Burkett*
- *3-3: Ethical Principles in Dental Hygiene—William Johnston*
- *3-4: Ethical Principles in Dental Hygiene—Maria Bjork*
- Review Portfolio Exercise 1-B.

Textbook
Review Case Study 3-1, Ethics and the Law, and Case Study 3-2, Ethical Decision Making Model, and the case applications.

Review the following:
- Box 3-3, Dental Hygiene Code of Ethics
- Box 3-4, Patient Bill of Rights

HOW do I perform these skills?

evolve
A printable version of this checklist is available on your Evolve Student Resources.
To comply with legal and ethical considerations, I will:
- ☐ Provide dental care in a manner that complies with the laws that govern my practice.
- ☐ Provide dental care following the professional code of ethics.
- ☐ Inform patient of goals to be achieved.
- ☐ Inform patient of therapy alternatives.
- ☐ Inform patient of the risks that may ensue from particular treatments.
- ☐ Inform patient of the risks that may ensue from no treatment.
- ☐ Obtain patient's written consent.
- ☐ Provide services in a manner that protects the patient and results in minimal harm.
- ☐ Document findings and procedure in chart.

HOW can I more effectively use this knowledge?

Critical Thinking Activities

1. In a small group of three to five students, review clinical case studies containing ethical and legal issues. Identify the nature of the ethical and legal issues, and discuss the process you would follow to handle these issues.
2. Obtain a dental hygiene plan from a clinical record or develop one. Role-play with a peer the presentation you would make to inform a patient of the procedures planned. Obtain consent to begin care.
3. Role-play the presentation of the patients' bill of rights, and ask peers to critique your presentation.
4. Review the patients' bill of rights developed for your dental hygiene program's clinic. Does it contain all the elements that should be included? If not, how would you improve it?
5. Critique informed consent documents obtained from various healthcare facilities.
6. Review your state's practice act, and discuss the role of the regulatory body in enforcing these laws.
7. Discuss the process used to introduce change to the practice act, either by the regulatory body or by another entity.

DO I have all the answers?

Review Questions

Check your answers against the Answer Key at the back of this Study Guide to assess what you have learned.

1. *Nonmaleficence* is the ethical principle that says a practitioner should
   a. Act in the best interest of the patient.
   b. Do no harm to the patient.
   c. Allow the patient to accept or reject treatment.
   d. Keep information about the patient's health status private.
2. Attempting to provide treatment to a patient that is beyond the training of a practitioner is a violation of which ethical principle?
   a. Veracity
   b. Competence
   c. Beneficence
   d. Nonmaleficence
3. Which of the following ethical principles gives the patient the right to be informed of the benefits and risks of treatment and to decide whether to accept the treatment?
   a. Veracity
   b. Paternalism
   c. Autonomy
   d. Confidentiality
4. The first step in the ethical decision-making model is to
   a. Collect information
   b. Identify the ethical dilemma
   c. State the options

d. Apply ethical principles
   e. Make the decision
5. Which one of the following describes the basis of informed consent?
   a. Protecting the dentist or dental hygienist from a lawsuit initiated by an angry patient
   b. Explaining the costs of dental care
   c. Reviewing the practitioner's credentials
   d. Providing the patient with all material facts regarding his or her proposed treatment
6. Which one of the following elements must be proven in court for a plaintiff to prevail on a tort claim?
   a. Mutual agreement, consideration, and breach
   b. Duty owed, breach of duty, harm, and causation
   c. Breach of duty
   d. Injuries and costs
7. Informed consent requires that a patient be told which one of the following?
   a. Alternative means of treatment
   b. Cost of treatment and alternatives
   c. Prognosis of treatment and alternatives
   d. Risks of treatment and alternatives
   e. All of the above
8. A patient's right to self-determination may be expressed as which one of the following?
   a. Patient's right to demand the treatment he or she wishes to receive
   b. Patient's right to direct his or her medical care
   c. Patient's right to participate in treatment choices
   d. None of the above
   e. All of the above
9. Thorough documentation of the treatment record should include which elements?
   a. Treatment provided
   b. Reason(s) treatment was provided
   c. How treatment was provided
   d. *a* and *b*
   e. All of the above
10. The practice of dental hygiene is affected by which one of the following laws?
    a. Statutory
    b. Common
    c. Federal
    d. Local
    e. All of the above
11. Which one of the following regulates dental hygiene in most states in the United States?
    a. State boards of dental hygiene
    b. Dental hygiene committees
    c. State boards of dentistry
    d. None of the above
12. Dental hygiene treatment should always be provided in a manner that _____ or _____ the standard of care.
    a. Equals; comes close to
    b. Meets; falls just below
    c. Is superior to; exceeds
    d. Meets; exceeds

13. The dental hygienist discusses a patient's assessment results with another dental hygienist in the office, but one who is not involved in the care of the patient. The dental hygienist may be liable for which one of the following?
    a. Failure to disclose
    b. Breach of confidentiality
    c. Failure to obtain informed consent
    d. Falling below the standard of care

WHERE do I go for more information or support?

evolve

For suggested web sites and agencies, additional readings and resources, and more chapter-specific information, please consult your Evolve Student Resources. Because of the ever-changing nature of the Internet, please keep in mind that web sites listed and their content may change.

CD-ROM

Reference files: As you work through the CD-ROM exercises, you should be able to print reference files and add them to your class materials. No specific reference files apply to this chapter.

HOW can I keep track of my progress toward competence?

As an ongoing picture of progress, record and monitor clinical experiences relating to Chapter 3 content in your Portfolio. Review Portfolio exercise 1-B.

Self-Reflection

On a regular basis, review these experiences (with a faculty member). Identify strengths, weaknesses (not just numbers), and changes that you would incorporate into your clinical care plan now that you have had these experiences.

4 Evidence-Based Decision Making

WHY do I need to know about Evidence-Based Decision Making?

The decisions made about clinical care must incorporate the best available scientific evidence to maximize the potential for successful patient care outcomes. Because practitioners rely on the publication of findings from well-designed research studies, the scientific literature is an essential tool for making evidence-based decisions to solve problems. This chapter defines the basic concepts and skills that enable dental hygiene practitioners to find, evaluate, and incorporate effectively the evidence and to access resources that are available to help advance evidence-based decision-making (EBDM) skills.

WHAT will I be able to do with this knowledge?

1. Define evidence-based decision making.
2. Discuss the principles of evidence-based decision making.
3. Explain the need for evidence-based decision making.
4. Identify the five steps and skills necessary to practice evidence-based decision making.
5. Discuss the benefits of evidence-based decision making.
6. Implement the evidence-based decision-making process.

HOW do I prepare myself to transfer this knowledge to patient care?

 Go to Chapter 4 content on your CD-ROM or search for "Literature."

CD Exercises

- *4-1: Purpose and Definition of Evidence-Based Decision Making:* Identify the EBDM principles.
- *4-2: Step 1: Asking Good Questions—PICO Process:* Identify the PICO process.
- *4-3: Levels of Evidence:* Order the level of evidence.
- *4-4: Where to Look—Internet Resources:* Review Internet resources.
- *4-5: Where to Look—PubMed:* Review PubMed instructions.
- *4-6: Where to Look—Web Sites:* Review dentally focused web sites.

Portfolio Features

- *4-A: Where to Look—PubMed:* Provides first exposure to PubMed, Internet resources, search engines, web sites, literature search, and dental Internet sites; introduces the Internet as a source for information and links to search engines, PubMed, and dentally-focused web sites; and provides a tutorial on how to locate a specific topic and instructions on how to do a literature search on PubMed.

Textbook

Review Case Study 4-1, Comparison of In-Office and At-Home Bleaching Techniques, and the case applications. Complete the following exercise regarding Case Study 4-1 at the beginning of the chapter.

Identify the four PICO components as presented in Case Study 4-1:

P = _____

I = _____

C = _____

O = _____

HOW do I perform these skills?

evolve

A printable version of this checklist is available on your Evolve Student Resources.

To apply the EBDM process accurately, I will:

☐ Convert information needs and problems into clinical questions so that they can be answered.

☐ Conduct a computerized search with maximal efficiency for finding the best external evidence with which to answer the question.

☐ Critically appraise the evidence for its validity and usefulness (clinical applicability).

☐ Apply the results of the appraisal, or evidence, in clinical practice.

☐ Evaluate the process and my performance.

HOW can I more effectively use this knowledge?

Critical Thinking Activities

Use the following worksheet to complete activity #6.

1. Identify questions raised when providing patient care to which you do not have an answer. Apply the evidence-based decision-making (EBDM) process by formulating a good question, conducting an efficient computerized search, critically appraising the evidence, applying the results in clinical practice, and evaluating the outcomes.
2. Develop PICO questions to compare the effectiveness of the two different medications or products (e.g., mouth rinses, adjunctive therapies) or to compare the effectiveness of two different procedures (e.g., hand and ultrasonic scaling compared with hand scaling alone).
3. Use the PICO process to develop a topic for a table clinic or poster presentation.
4. Complete the PubMed tutorial to learn how to perform an effective database search.
5. Visit the Cochrane Library web site, and explore the different research groups and the available systematic reviews related to dental hygiene treatment, preventive procedures, and tobacco cessation.
6. Observe an appointment procedure with a classmate. Using Worksheet #1, evaluate for evidence of PICO during a patient education encounter.

Worksheet #1

Record your findings from Critical Thinking Activity #6 in this table.

Student	PICO	Topic	Evaluation and Remarks
#1	P		
	I		
	C		
	O		
#2	P		
	I		
	C		
	O		
#3	P		
	I		
	C		
	O		
#4	P		
	I		
	C		
	O		
#5	P		
	I		
	C		
	O		

DO I have all the answers?

Review Questions

Check your answers against the Answer Key at the back of this Study Guide to assess what you have learned.

Place the letter of the following steps in the EBDM process in the correct order *(the first through the fifth steps)*:

1. _____ a. Finding the best evidence
2. _____ b. Applying the results to patient care
3. _____ c. Asking a good clinical question
4. _____ d. Evaluating the results
5. _____ e. Critically appraising the evidence
6. Which one of the following elements demonstrates that EBDM has come of age?
   a. American Dental Association (ADA) accreditation standards for dental education
   b. American Dental Education Association (ADEA) competencies for dental and dental hygiene education
   c. Evidence-based journals
   d. ADA has defined EBDM
   e. All of the above
7. Which one of the following reasons has *not* contributed to the need for EBDM?
   a. Variations in practice patterns
   b. Delays in adopting useful procedures
   c. Increased access to relevant clinical findings
   d. Practicing as taught in school
   e. Providing effective patient care
8. Which one of the following research designs provides the highest level of evidence?
   a. Animal study
   b. Case control study
   c. Cohort study
   d. Laboratory study
   e. Randomized controlled trial

Match the following characteristics with the type of publication:

Literature review *(a)* or Systematic review *(b)*

_____ 9. Specific problem or patient question
_____ 10. Conducted by one person versus a team
_____ 11. Broad focus
_____ 12. Identification of databases searched
_____ 13. Includes studies determined at the reviewer's discretion
_____ 14. Statistical analysis of the data

15. Match the terms with the most appropriate PICO component:

_____ P a. Treatment under consideration
_____ I b. Main concern or chief complaint
_____ C c. Measurable result
_____ O d. Alternative treatment

WHERE do I go for more information or support?

evolve

For suggested web sites and agencies, additional readings and resources, and more chapter-specific information, please consult your Evolve Student Resources. Because of the ever-changing nature of the Internet, please keep in mind that web sites listed and their content may change.

CD CD-ROM

Reference files: As you work through the CD-ROM exercises, you should be able to print reference files and add them to your class materials. No specific reference files apply to this chapter.

HOW can I keep track of my progress toward competence?

As an ongoing picture of progress, record and monitor clinical experiences relating to Chapter 4 content in your Portfolio.

Self-Reflection

On a regular basis, review these experiences (with a faculty member). Identify strengths, weaknesses (not just numbers), and changes that you would incorporate into your clinical care plan now that you have had these experiences.

5 Communication

WHY do I need to know about Communication?

Effective communication skills are vital to excellent patient care. Although a dental hygienist may have good clinical skills, when the professional is unable to communicate effectively with the patient through verbal and nonverbal mechanisms, the overall experience for the patient will be limited.

WHAT will I be able to do with this knowledge?

1. Recognize that effective communication skills can be learned.
2. Identify the stages in the acquisition of new skills: knowledge, interest, belief, commitment, practice, and habituation.
3. Distinguish among the three key attributes to effective communication: listening, observing, and attending.
4. Explain the function of space, time, culture, context, and language in the establishment of rapport.
5. Identify and explain the importance of core nonverbal behaviors such as facial expression, body language, and eye contact.
6. Explain and demonstrate key elements of deepening rapport: empathy, respect, warmth, concreteness, genuineness, and self-disclosure.
7. Become a better communicator by providing positive feedback, using "I" messages, and practicing active listening.
8. Evaluate with discernment the principles of communication.
9. Explain how a patient's behavioral style influences the communication process.

HOW do I prepare myself to transfer this knowledge to patient care?

 Go to Chapter 5 content on your CD-ROM or search for "Patient Communication."

CD Exercises

- *5-1: Key Elements of Communication—Terrence Zellar—Video:* Determine principles of communication from the video.
- *5-2: Understanding Behavioral Styles:* Match the behavioral characteristics to the four types.

- *5-3: Understanding Behavioral Styles—Strategies:* Match the behavioral type and the communication strategy based on patient scenario.
- *5-4: Key Elements of Communication—Terrence Zellar*
- *5-5 to 5-6: Key Elements of Communication—Terrence Zellar—Video:* Determine principles of communication from the video.
- *5-7: Key Elements of Communication—Audio:* Answer questions from a telephone call regarding smoking information.

Textbook

Review Case Study 5-1, Team Approach to Communication, and the case applications.

HOW do I perform these skills?

evolve

A printable version of this checklist is available on your Evolve Student Resources.
To communicate effectively during patient care, I will:
- ☐ Actively listen to the patient's thoughts and concerns.
- ☐ Observe the patient with warmth and empathy while making eye contact.
- ☐ Attend to the patient.
- ☐ Establish patient rapport.
- ☐ Maintain a comfortable distance from the patient.
- ☐ Recognize and understand cultural differences.
- ☐ Use context appropriately.
- ☐ Use time effectively.
- ☐ Communicate using appropriate language.
- ☐ Observe patient for nonverbal cues.
- ☐ Provide positive feedback when appropriate.

HOW can I more effectively use this knowledge?

Critical Thinking Activities

Use the following worksheets to complete activity #2.
1. Using Case Study 5-1, identify the effective elements of communication that Andrea used during her interaction with Mr. McPherson.

2. Using personal encounters, reflect on your own communication style. Using Worksheet #1, keep a journal for several days, and identify the specific occasions when you demonstrated effective elements of communication. In addition, identify the barriers in the maintenance of effective communication skills.
3. Write a composite of the communication skills that you would look for if you were a dentist hiring a dental hygienist for a full-time position in a private practice dental office.
4. Observe a senior dental hygienist while he or she is providing services to a patient. List the nonverbal forms of communication used by both the dental hygiene student and the patient.
5. Conduct an interview with a geriatric patient while a fellow student observes you. The interview should include a thorough medical, dental, and social history. The peer observer should record all verbal and nonverbal elements of communication that enhanced the interview, in addition to those elements that served as a barrier for effective communication.
6. Select a periodontally involved patient, and provide oral hygiene instruction while a classmate videotapes the session. Critique your own communication style, and identify areas that can be changed to enhance your communication effectiveness.

Worksheet #1

Record your findings from Critical Thinking Activity #2 on this form. Identify at least one communication experience per day for 1 week. At the end of the day, complete the self-assessment form. Remember that effective communication is dynamic; messages and images flow between the sender and receiver. Both verbal and nonverbal actions are important to outcomes.

	Communication Event	Effective Elements	Barrier or Barriers
Day 1			
Day 2			
Day 3			
Day 4			
Day 5			
Day 6			
Day 7			

Worksheet #2

Using this listing and your textbook as references, identify which of the communication elements listed were used successfully in Critical Thinking Activity #2.

Key Elements of Communication	More Successful	Less Successful
Listening	☐	☐
Observing	☐	☐
Establishing rapport	☐	☐
Regulating verbal communication	☐	☐
Reflecting interest in the discussion	☐	☐
Expressing emotion	☐	☐
Conveying status and describing personal characteristics	☐	☐
Expressing warmth	☐	☐
Being direct	☐	☐
Being concrete	☐	☐
Being genuine	☐	☐
Self-disclosure	☐	☐
Using the "I" message	☐	☐

DO I have all the answers?

Review Questions

Check your answers against the Answer Key at the back of this Study Guide to assess what you have learned.

1. Dr. Marian Jones, a dentist, is discussing the treatment plan with her patient, Bill Truman. The patient states, "Do I really need the periodontal surgery that you are describing, Dr. Jones?" Which of the following responses by Dr. Jones would demonstrate *reflective listening?*
   a. "Yes, Mr. Truman, you already know the answer to that question."
   b. "Are you nervous, Mr. Truman?"
   c. "Yes, Mr. Truman, but don't worry, it won't be a painful procedure."
   d. "Mr. Truman, you seem to be concerned about the surgery."

2. Laura Buffington, a patient, is discussing her oral hygiene practices with her dental hygienist, Teresa. Ms. Buffington laments that she has been trying hard to floss on a regular basis but cannot seem to get to it everyday as Teresa has advised. Which one of the following responses by Teresa would demonstrate *empathy?*
   a. "Two or three times a week? You'll have to do better than that, Ms. Buffington."
   b. "You'll lose your teeth, Ms. Buffington, if you don't start flossing every day."
   c. "Ms. Buffington, that's a great start. I know it's hard to fit flossing into your schedule."
   d. "Don't blame me, Ms. Buffington, when Dr. Blank tells you that you'll need surgery."

3. Effective listening is a passive process. Effective communication involves participation by both the sender and the receiver of the message.
   a. Both statements are true.
   b. Both statements are false.
   c. The first statement is true; the second statement is false.
   d. The first statement is false; the second statement is true.

4. "Dr. Gonzalez, I am not comfortable charging Mr. Hartrick's insurance company for quadrant scaling when he does not need it. I believe that it is wrong to submit insurance claims for treatment that is not indicated. I would like to schedule Mr. Hartrick for a maintenance 6-month prophylaxis." Kim, the dental hygienist, was demonstrating which communication skill?
   a. Empathy
   b. Providing feedback using "I" statements
   c. Paraphrasing
   d. Genuineness
   e. Both *b* and *d* are correct.

WHERE do I go for more information or support?

evolve

For suggested web sites and agencies, additional readings and resources, and more chapter-specific information, please consult your Evolve Student Resources. Because of the ever-changing nature of the Internet, please keep in mind that web sites listed and their content may change.

CD-ROM

Reference files: As you work through the CD-ROM exercises, you should be able to print reference files and add them to your class materials. No specific reference files apply to this chapter.

HOW can I keep track of my progress toward competence?

As an ongoing picture of progress, record and monitor clinical experiences relating to Chapter 5 content in your Portfolio.

Self-Reflection

On a regular basis, review these experiences (with a faculty member). Identify strengths, weaknesses (not just numbers), and changes that you would incorporate into your clinical care plan now that you have had these experiences.

6 The Body's Response to Challenge

WHY do I need to know about The Body's Response to Challenge?

The body is continually exposed to a variety of microbes, many of which are normally found in the body and others that pose a significant threat for causing infection and disease. The human body is capable of responding to these threats with a variety of complex, highly regulated processes that allow the body to rid itself of invaders and resultant infections and by facilitating repair. This chapter reviews the processes of inflammation, immune response, hemostasis, and wound healing. Normal events, as well as alterations in response and associated pathophysiology, are also discussed. Understanding these concepts is essential for the dental hygienist because these topics make up the framework of host response mechanisms critical for function and survival.

WHAT will I be able to do with this knowledge?

1. Describe the function of each type of white blood cell.
2. Correlate the cardinal signs of inflammation with the vascular and cellular changes associated with the inflammatory process.
3. Compare the histopathologic characteristics associated with acute and chronic inflammation.
4. Discuss the physiologic effects of the chemicals that mediate the inflammatory response.
5. Describe the host response mechanisms of innate immunity.
6. Describe the host response mechanisms of adaptive immunity.
7. Discuss the role of cellular specificity and memory in immune response.
8. Describe the immunoglobulins associated with immune response and allergic reactions.
9. Describe the clinical signs and symptoms associated with hypersensitivity reactions.
10. Discuss the mechanisms of clot formation and hemostasis.
11. Contrast healing by primary versus secondary intention.
12. Discuss the etiology of adverse thromboembolic events and the appropriate interventions used to reduce the associated complications.

HOW do I prepare myself to transfer this knowledge to patient care?

Go to Chapter 6 content on your CD-ROM or search for "Immune System."

CD Exercises

- *6-1: Key Terms:* Match key terms to definitions in the chapter.
- *6-2: Inflammatory Events:* Order the events in the inflammatory responses correctly and view an animation of the process.
- *6-3: Stages of Immune Response:* Order the five stages of the immune response.

Textbook

Review Case Study 6-1, New Patient Indicates Allergy to Novocaine, and the case applications. Start answering the following questions regarding Case Study 6-1:
a. Have any adverse reactions occurred that he or she has experienced related to medication use or other substances known to trigger these reactions?
b. Is noting that patients experience food allergies important? Why?
c. Should patients with allergies to preservatives, including the sulfites, be contraindicated for use of dental local anesthetics?
   - What are the clinical signs and symptoms described by the patient?
   - Was medical intervention necessary at the time of the reaction? What was the time between exposure and onset of symptoms? Were any medications used to reverse the reaction?

HOW can I more effectively use this knowledge?

Critical Thinking Activities

1. Examine a patient with periodontal disease, and correlate the clinical signs and symptoms with the stages of the inflammatory response. Based on the clinical appearance of the tissues, determine whether the inflammation is acute or chronic in nature.
2. Identify the drugs in the dental office emergency kit that are used to treat adverse events associated with abnormal bleeding and allergic reactions. Discuss how

each of these agents affects the symptoms in question and their proposed mechanisms of action.

3. Request a copy of the laboratory test results used to evaluate coagulation in a patient taking oral anticoagulant therapy. Interpret the test results to determine whether it is safe to provide dental hygiene care. Determine the need for modifications in the dental hygiene treatment plan as a result of the test results.

4. Monitor the course of healing time in a patient with sutures after periodontal surgery, as compared with a patient healing from third molar extraction surgery. Describe the course of events related to healing in terms of time, tissue appearance, and any complications associated with both surgeries. Discuss strategies that could be used to minimize complications associated with these surgical procedures.

DO I have all the answers?

Review Questions

Check your answers against the Answer Key at the back of this Study Guide to assess what you have learned.

1. Which one of the following best describes the primary function of granulocytes and monocytes?
   a. Tissue repair
   b. Phagocytosis
   c. Antigen-antibody binding
   d. Opsonization

2. Which one of the following white blood cells increases production as a result of parasitic infections?
   a. Lymphocytes
   b. Monocytes
   c. Neutrophils
   d. Eosinophils

3. Which one of the following cell types is primarily responsible for the secretion of histamine?
   a. Neutrophil
   b. Eosinophil
   c. Mast cell
   d. Activated T lymphocyte

4. Which process best describes the white blood cells exiting the blood vessels through the pores?
   a. Margination
   b. Pavementing
   c. Diapedesis
   d. Opsonization

5. Which one of the following clinical conditions results from uncontrolled production of white blood cells?
   a. Leukemia
   b. Leukopenia
   c. Leukocytosis
   d. Leukocytis

6. Which one of the following processes is responsible for the unidirectional movement by neutrophils and macrophages to the site of inflammation?
   a. Diapedesis
   b. Opsonization
   c. Chemotaxis
   d. Phagocytosis

7. Which one of the following processes is responsible for edema associated with inflammation?
   a. Vasodilation
   b. Increased vascular permeability
   c. White blood cell migration
   d. Phagocytosis

8. Which one of the following is responsible for the initiation of cellular signaling mechanisms and the regulation of growth proliferation and maturation of cells?
   a. Cytokines
   b. Hormones
   c. Growth factors
   d. Kinins

9. Which one of the following complement proteins acts as a chemoattractant for white blood cells?
   a. C3a
   b. C3b
   c. C4a
   d. C5a

10. Which one of the following conditions increases the production and release of leukotrienes?
    a. Asthma
    b. Arthritis
    c. Thromboembolic disorders
    d. Pain

11. Which one of the following actions best describes the role of T lymphocytes?
    a. Produces antibodies
    b. Recognizes and destroys antigens from foreign sources
    c. Mediates humoral immunity
    d. Attacks host cells

12. Which one of the following processes can be attributed to the ability of the immune system to distinguish between millions of different types of antigens or portions of antigens?
    a. T-cell activation
    b. B-cell activation
    c. Cellular specificity
    d. Cellular memory

13. Which one of the following events results from repeated exposure to an antigen?
    a. Same immune reaction
    b. Heightened immune reaction
    c. Diminished immune reaction
    d. Self-tolerance

14. Which one of the following clotting pathways is activated when trauma to the wall of a blood vessel or the surrounding tissue has occurred?
    a. Immunoglobulin A (IgA)
    b. Immunoglobulin E (IgE)
    c. Immunoglobulin G (IgG)
    d. Immunoglobulin M (IgM)

15. Trauma to the wall of a blood vessel or the surrounding tissue results in activation of which of the following clotting pathways?
    a. Extrinsic
    b. Intrinsic

16. The use of sutures to close a wound promotes healing through which of the following intentions?
    a. Primary
    b. Secondary

WHERE do I go for more information or support?

For suggested web sites and agencies, additional readings and resources, and more chapter-specific information, please consult your Evolve Student Resources. Because of the ever-changing nature of the Internet, please keep in mind that web sites listed and their content may change.

CD-ROM

Reference files: As you work through the CD-ROM exercises, you should be able to print reference files and add them to your class materials. No specific reference files apply to this chapter.

HOW can I keep track of my progress toward competence?

As an ongoing picture of progress, record and monitor clinical experiences relating to Chapter 6 content in your Portfolio.

Self-Reflection

On a regular basis, review these experiences (with a faculty member). Identify strengths, weaknesses (not just numbers), and changes that you would incorporate into your clinical care plan now that you have had these experiences.

7 Exposure Control and Prevention of Disease Transmission

WHY do I need to know about Exposure Control and Prevention of Disease Transmission?

The dental hygiene professional has the ethical responsibility to integrate many principles into practice: basic science, principles of safety, and professional standards of care and policy, as well as to comply with numerous federal, state, and local regulations applied to infection control in the healthcare setting. Once this responsibility is understood, dental hygienists then must provide their patients oral healthcare services in a way that protects the health of both the patients and the dental healthcare personnel.

WHAT will I be able to do with this knowledge?

1. State the basic principles and science of disease transmission and common infectious diseases of humans, infection control in the dental workplace, and safety as it applies to biohazards in the dental workplace.
2. Identify the names of state and federal regulatory and advisory agencies that concern infection control practices and the management of biohazardous materials.
3. Integrate basic science, clinical practice, professional standards of care, and regulatory standards for infection control and work-practice safety to prevent disease transmission and protect the health of both employees and patients in the dental workplace.
4. Apply effective principles of infection control and safe handling of biohazardous materials to provide a safe environment for dental hygienists, co-workers, patients in the dental workplace, and household members.
5. Comply with federal, state, and local standards and regulations for the dental workplace.

HOW do I prepare myself to transfer this knowledge to patient care?

 Go to Chapter 7 content on your CD-ROM or search for "Infection Control."

CD Exercises
- *7-1: Standard Precautions:* Determine requirements.
- *7-2: Personal Protective Equipment (PPE):* Select appropriate PPE for various functions.
- *7-3: Environmental Surface Protection:* Select appropriate disinfection procedures at beginning of the day.
- *7-4: Environmental Surface Protection:* Select appropriate disinfection procedures between appointments.
- *7-5: Sterilization—Video:* Watch video clip.
- *7-6: Sterilization: Instrument Processing:* Place the steps for steam sterilization procedure in the correct order.
- *7-7: Waste Management:* Select correct waste management.
- *7-8: Waste Management—Audio:* Respond to a patient's infection control concerns from a telephone call.

Textbook
Review Case Study 7-1 through 7-4 and the case applications.

For important concepts and application of knowledge, the following text elements may be especially helpful for clinical transfer and may be used as a clinical resource:
- Tables 7-1 and 7-5 through 7-7
- Box 7-2
- Figures 7-4 through 7-8, 7-10, and 7-12 through 7-15

HOW do I perform these skills?

evolve

A printable version of this checklist is available on your Evolve Student Resources.

To comply with OSHA standards, I will perform the following:

Prepare for Patient Treatment
- ☐ Use all appropriate PPE.
- ☐ Gather all necessary supplies, and organize them in the treatment room according to the work zones defined for that workspace.
- ☐ Flush water lines.
- ☐ Use surface barriers, as appropriate.

Demonstrate Proper Treatment Room Cleanup
- ☐ Use proper PPE for operator.
- ☐ Ensure that all instruments and equipment are safely transported for processing.
- ☐ Properly dispose of waste.
- ☐ Remove all disposable barriers.
- ☐ Disinfect any surfaces that are visibly contaminated with blood, have been touched, or may have been contaminated during treatment.

29

Demonstrate Proper Instrument Processing

☐ Use proper PPE for operator.
☐ Place instruments in ultrasonic (cleaner).
☐ Rinse and pat dry as indicated.
☐ Appropriately package instruments according to the sterilization process used.
☐ Sterilize instruments.
☐ Store instruments.
☐ Replace barriers.
☐ Flush water lines.

At the End of Day

☐ Remove all surface barriers.
☐ Use the *spray-wipe-spray* procedure to disinfect treatment room.
☐ Flush the evacuation system.

HOW can I more effectively use this knowledge?

Critical Thinking Activities

Use the following worksheet to complete activity #5.

1. Review Case Study 7-1 about Ruth, the dental office manager. Remember that Ruth's primary duties are at the front desk, although she occasionally helps when the staff is behind schedule. Ruth's duties require that she regularly handle patient charts, filing, and billing and insurance papers. Often, she is the first person to receive the patient chart at the completion of the appointment.

   Ruth has missed several weeks of work and is showing lingering signs of a systemic illness. She may have contracted an illness at work. Using this knowledge, address the following issues:
   a. Review her work responsibilities and determine whether she is considered at high risk for occupational transmission.
   b. Which tasks would place her at risk?
   c. Is she at risk from the work practices of others in the office?
   d. Which OSHA abatement strategies would reduce the previously stated risks?

2. Review Case Study 7-2 about the dental hygiene student in her second (final) year. If you had been the student who noticed that the cycle integrator on the sterilization bag had not changed for the instruments you had used, which steps would you need to take to identify which load or loads of instruments had been distributed without the indication that appropriate sterilization had taken place?

   You have determined that the instruments appear to have been used during a student laboratory session, and some have been used on patients in the general clinic. At least one patient is confirmed to have been exposed to unsterilized instruments, but no other students are able to confirm whether the instruments they used in their session were from the same load. Review the standard operating procedures (SOPs) for your sterilization area, given the same incident, and answer the following questions:
   a. Could you determine the following?
      1. How many packs must be found? How many were sterilized in the batches in question?
      2. How many packs were opened and used?
      3. For which patients or activities were the packs used?
      4. Which procedures would assist you in determining on whom the instruments in question were used?
   b. If you are unable to follow up on tasks 1 through 4, then develop a SOP that would allow you to track the loads in question.

3. Review Case Study 7-3 about the dental hygienist wiping an instrument to clean the tip. Think about times in which you have observed a dental hygienist withdraw an instrument from a patient's mouth with a significant mass of blood and debris adhered to the working end. Without thinking, many hygienists reach over with a pinching motion and wipe the instrument clean with a piece of gauze. Consider the following issues:
   a. Discuss the risks involved in wiping instruments in your fingers.
   b. Examine resources in your clinic, and develop a hands-free method to debride your instrument during patient treatment.
   c. Present an argument in favor of the implementation of safer work practice controls (WPCs).

4. Review Case Study 7-4 about Mr. Birdwell, and reflect on his activities before he developed the eye infection:
   a. Do you agree with the probable cause of his infection?
   b. Which OSHA WPCs would provide protection from this incident in the future?
   c. Are safeguards in place in your clinic to prevent such an incident?
   d. Which SOPs could be implemented to prevent a repeat occurrence?

5. Using Worksheet #1, observe 5 classmates during an appointed procedure. Evaluate for infection control risks, determine the appropriate corrective action, and identify your clinic policy on the subject.

Worksheet #1

Record your findings from Critical Thinking Activity #5 in this table.

Classmate	Infection Control Risk	Corrective Action	Clinic Policy
#1			
#2			
#3			
#4			
#5			

Chapter **7** **Exposure Control and Prevention of Disease Transmission**

Review Questions

Check your answers against the Answer Key at the back of this Study Guide to assess what you have learned.

1. An infection resulting from the introduction of microorganisms from one area of the body to another occurs via which one of the following methods of transmission?
   a. Autogenous
   b. Aerosol
   c. Direct
   d. Indirect
2. Which one of the following factors is the most important in the development of an infection within a host?
   a. The dose of the pathogenic microorganisms transmitted
   b. The integrity of the host's immune system
   c. The virulence of the microorganisms transmitted
   d. All of the above have significant influence on the development of disease; one factor cannot be singled out.
3. Which of the following diseases is caused by bacterial agents?
   a. Candidiasis, hepatitis, legionella
   b. Legionella, pneumonia, tuberculosis
   c. Influenza, pneumonia, tuberculosis
   d. Candidiasis, legionella, tuberculosis
4. You have purchased some instrument trays for use in the office that are made of heat-sensitive plastic, and the following label was included in the package:

Dental Set-Up Tray

To Sterilize:
Use alcohol or other approved disinfectants.

   Which of the following statements is correct?
   a. Instructions provided are correct. Sterilization of the tray would be accomplished.
   b. Instructions provided are partially correct. Sterilization of the tray would be accomplished with the use of alcohol but not with other approved disinfectants.
   c. Instructions provided are partially correct. Sterilization of the tray would be accomplished with other approved disinfectants but not with alcohol.
   d. Instructions provided are incorrect. Sterilization of the tray would be not be accomplished by either method listed.

5. OSHA has defined which one of the following as primary hazard abatement strategies to reduce the risk of occupational exposures to blood-borne diseases?
   a. Universal controls (UC), housekeeping, and engineering precautions (EP)
   b. Universal precautions (UP), personal protective engineering (PPE), and labels
   c. Universal precautions (UP), work practice controls (WPC), and record keeping
   d. Universal controls (UC), personal protective equipment (PPE), and training

WHERE do I go for more information or support?

evolve

For suggested web sites and agencies, additional readings and resources, and more chapter-specific information, please consult your Evolve Student Resources. Because of the ever-changing nature of the Internet, please keep in mind that web sites listed and their content may change.

 CD-ROM

Reference files: As you work through the CD-ROM exercises, you should be able to print reference files and add them to your class materials. No specific reference files apply to this chapter.

HOW can I keep track of my progress toward competence?

As an ongoing picture of progress, record and monitor clinical experiences relating to Chapter 7 content in your Portfolio.

Self-Reflection

On a regular basis, review these experiences (with a faculty member). Identify strengths, weaknesses (not just numbers), and changes that you would incorporate into your clinical care plan now that you have had these experiences.

8 Positioning and Prevention of Operator Injury

WHY do I need to know about Positioning and Prevention of Operator Injury?

Learning and adapting ergonomic positioning and practices is critical for physical comfort, proper muscle tone, and reduction of musculoskeletal challenges of the dental hygienist. The benefits of good posture and performance-logic positioning during dental hygiene procedures are fundamental to establishing and maintaining musculoskeletal health.

WHAT will I be able to do with this knowledge?

1. Develop an appreciation for evidence-based knowledge of ergonomics in the dental environment.
2. Understand the relationship among correct operator posture and positioning, patient and equipment positioning, and musculoskeletal problems.
3. Describe the physical changes that occur from repetitive strain injuries.
4. Demonstrate correct operator, patient, and equipment positioning for maximal efficiency and minimal risk of developing musculoskeletal problems.
5. Compare, contrast, and evaluate alternative operator and patient positions.
6. Correct improper positioning by recognizing cues that indicate that an aspect of positioning is incorrect.
7. Develop an awareness of new technology that may reduce operator stress and fatigue and promote optimal performance.
8. Incorporate preventive exercises into instrumentation procedures.
9. Perform preventive exercises throughout the workday and at home.
10. Apply correct operator, patient, and equipment positioning for maximal efficiency for ultrasonic scaling.

HOW do I prepare myself to transfer this knowledge to patient care?

 Go to Chapter 8 content on your CD-ROM or search for "Ergonomics."

CD Exercises

- *8-1 and 8-2: Ergonomics Associated with Dental Hygiene Practice:* Given two specific clinical scenarios, determine the type of repetitive strain disorder outcome.
- *8-3: Positioning:* Identify specific operator and patient positioning errors.

Textbook

Review Case Study 8-1, Musculoskeletal Problems Resulting from Equipment, and the case applications.

For important concepts and application of knowledge, the following text elements may be especially helpful for clinical transfer and may be used as a clinical resource:
- Table 8-1
- Boxes 8-1 through 8-6
- Figures 8-13 through 8-29

HOW do I perform these skills?

evolve

A printable version of this checklist is available on your Evolve Student Resources.
To apply body ergonomics in the dental care setting, I will perform the following:

Practice Operator Positioning

- ☐ Sit tall in the chair with legs separated.
- ☐ Place thighs parallel to the floor.
- ☐ Place feet flat on the floor.
- ☐ Traditional approach: Work from 8 to 12 o'clock; Performance logic approach: Work within the range of 10 and 12 o'clock.
- ☐ Place equipment as close to the operator as possible to avoid excessive bending or twisting.
- ☐ Keep elbows in a relaxed position and near sides.
- ☐ Maintain wrists in a neutral position.

Practice Patient Positioning

- ☐ Keep patient in the supine position throughout the appointment.
- ☐ Position overhead light directly into the patient's oral cavity, avoiding shadows.

HOW can I more effectively use this knowledge?

Critical Thinking Activities

Use the following worksheet to complete activity #6.

1. Practice the exercises described in the "Postural Exercises" section in Chapter 8 of *Mosby's Dental Hygiene, 2nd Edition.*
2. Find the head of the fibula, and determine the correct height for the operator chair.
3. Using the performance-logic position, correctly position the following:
   a. Yourself in the operator chair
   b. Student partner in the dental chair
   c. Equipment to work on the mandibular arch (Ask the student partner to turn his or her head toward the operator.)

Attempt to activate an exploratory stroke on the mandibular left lingual. Can you as the operator see? Does this feel correct? Next, ask the student partner to turn his or her head slightly away from you. Can you see? Does it feel correct? Is there a shadow cast on the arch? Is it possible to activate a stroke without struggling? What positions are incorrect? Was your ability to activate the stroke improved?

4. Determine your own balanced reference point as described in Boxes 8-2 and 8-3.
5. Practice traditional patient and operator positioning, and work in the same areas as described in question 3.
6. Using Worksheet #1, observe the posture and positioning of another dental hygiene student, and identify correct and incorrect postures and positions.

Worksheet #1

Working in groups of three—one evaluator, one patient, and one clinician—evaluate and provide feedback for proper patient positioning. Space is provided for the area for which the patient is being positioned for best visibility and instrumentation. Both the patient and the evaluator should provide feedback; roles should be switched until each student has served in all three roles. Record your findings from Critical Thinking Activity #6 on this worksheet.

Area of Instrumentation	Feedback

Patient Positioning

Supine position (feet and head on same plane) _____

Semisupine position (medical or musculoskeletal problems) _____

Patient nose level with clinician heart _____

Maxillary Instrumentation

Occlusal plane perpendicular to floor _____

Head rotated in appropriate direction for area being worked on _____

Mandibular Instrumentation

Occlusal plane parallel to floor _____

Head rotated in appropriate direction for area being worked on _____

Range of Position

10:00-12:30 maintained (right hand) _____

2:00-11:30 maintained (left hand) _____

Light

Maxillary Arch

Directly above patient's chest _____

Mandibular Arch

Directly above patient's head _____

Arm's length from operator (at 36 inches) _____

DO I have all the answers?

Review Questions

Check your answers against the Answer Key at the back of this Study Guide to assess what you have learned.
Question 1 refers to Case Study 8-1.

1. Which one of the following is the most likely cause for the development of Suzanne's musculoskeletal problems?
   a. Improper instrumentation positioning
   b. Improper patient positioning
   c. Improper positioning of the dental equipment
   d. Improper chair height

2. In McKenzie's classification system, which one of the following syndromes is the most difficult to treat?
   a. Derangement syndrome
   b. Postural syndrome
   c. Dysfunction syndrome

3. Physiologically, which one of the following describes the number of normal curves in the human spine?
   a. Two
   b. Three
   c. One
   d. Four

4. The human spine has two normal lordosis curves and two normal kyphosis curves.
   a. The first part of the sentence is true, and the second part is false.
   b. Both parts of the sentence are true.
   c. Both parts of the sentence are false.
   d. The first part of the sentence is false, and the second is true.

5. Which one of the following describes the recommended distance of the operator's head to the patient's oral cavity?
   a. 6 to 8 inches
   b. 8 to 10 inches
   c. 12 to 14 inches
   d. It does not matter as long as the operator is comfortable.

6. The dental light should be approximately how many inches from the oral cavity?
   a. 12
   b. 18
   c. 24
   d. 36

7. Which one of the following describes performance-logic positioning?
   a. Proprioceptive derivation
   b. Reduces work-related musculoskeletal disorders
   c. Decreases operator repositioning
   d. All of the above

WHERE do I go for more information or support?

evolve

For suggested web sites and agencies, additional readings and resources, and more chapter-specific information, please consult your Evolve Student Resources. Because of the ever-changing nature of the Internet, please keep in mind that web sites listed and their content may change.

CD-ROM

Reference files: As you work through the CD-ROM exercises, you should be able to print reference files and add them to your class materials. No specific reference files apply to this chapter.

HOW can I keep track of my progress toward competence?

As an ongoing picture of progress, record and monitor clinical experiences relating to Chapter 8 content in your Portfolio.

Self-Reflection

On a regular basis, review these experiences (with a faculty member). Identify strengths, weaknesses (not just numbers), and changes that you would incorporate into your clinical care plan now that you have had these experiences.

9 Instrument Design and Principles of Instrumentation

WHY do I need to know about Instrument Design and Principles of Instrumentation?

Dental instruments are a basic component of intraoral evaluation and treatment. Complete knowledge and understanding of dental instruments and their design, function, and clinical applications make up the foundation of successful treatment outcomes. This complete understanding affords the clinician the critical thinking skills necessary to adapt appropriately and use successfully any dental instrument.

WHAT will I be able to do with this knowledge?

1. Identify instruments by classification, design name, and design number.
2. Describe the function of each part of any instrument.
3. Analyze each principle step by step as it relates to instrumentation.
4. Select the appropriate instrument by design based on the periodontal condition.
5. Demonstrate correct principles of instrumentation in preclinical and clinical sessions.
6. Compare and contrast the powered instrument design and principles of use with hand instruments in periodontal debridement.

HOW do I prepare myself to transfer this knowledge to patient care?

 Go to Chapter 9 content on your CD-ROM or search for "Instrumentation."

CD Exercises

- *9-1: Fundamentals of Instrumentation:* Identify the steps on instrumentation by rationale correctly.
- *9-2: Fundamentals of Instrumentation:* Define the steps in instrumentation using purpose and rationale correctly.
- *9-3: Activation—Video:* Once the correct type of activation stroke has been identified for each type of activation stroke, the video and animation will run.

Textbook

Review Case Study 9-1, Instrument Selection Evaluation, and the case applications.

For important concepts and application of knowledge, the following text elements may be especially helpful for clinical transfer and may be used as a clinical resource:

- Tables 9-1 through 9-3
- Box 9-2
- Figures 9-1 through 9-38

HOW do I perform these skills?

evolve

A printable version of this checklist is available on your Evolve Student Resources.

During instrument selection and implementation, I will:

☐ Select appropriate instrument by design based on periodontal condition.

☐ Use proper instrument grasp.

☐ Maintain proper fulcrum.

☐ Keep the working end against the tooth surface at all times.

☐ Close the face of the blade during subgingival insertion.

☐ Maintain the terminal shank parallel to the long axis of the tooth during instrumentation.

☐ Roll instrument handle between the index finger and thumb for adaptation.

☐ Pivot on the fulcrum finger.

☐ Maintain proper tooth-to-blade angulation during instrumentation.

☐ Initiate proper instrument activation.

HOW can I more effectively use this knowledge?

Critical Thinking Activities

Use the following worksheet to complete activity #5.

1. A fellow student has a tray set-up of various scaling instruments. She is asking for your assistance in identifying the various instruments by name, use, and location in the oral cavity. The set-up consists of curets, sickles, probes, explorers, and dental mirrors. Several specialty instruments such as files, chisels, and hoes are also included. Using knowledge of the design features for scaling instruments, help your colleague with instrument identification and use.

2. Now that the instruments have been identified, assist your classmate with instrument practice on the typodont. Observe the principles of instrumentation, and assist with skill development. Identify problems that can be

37

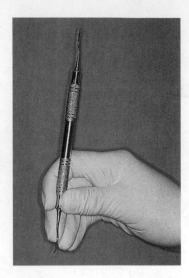
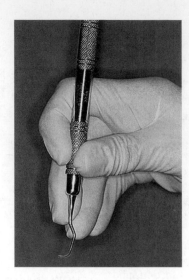
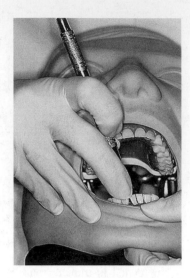

encountered, and develop suggestions to overcome the problem.

3. Examine the instrument grasp in the illustrations above. Determine the possible errors with each grasp and the technique errors that could result from an inappropriate grasp.

4. Using two dental mirrors, practice instrument grasp and fulcrum technique in the clinic with a student partner. Remove the mirror from one of the instruments. Holding the handle in the dominant hand, work on grasp, fulcrum, and pivoting in each sextant of the mouth.

5. Using Worksheet #1, create an identification test with instruments from your kit. Cover the design name and number, and try to identify the instrument and its location for use.

6. Practice instrumentation in groups of three in the clinic. One student serves as the operator, another as the patient, and the third as an evaluator. Using your instrument evaluation form, the evaluator will examine operator technique for strengths and weaknesses. The patient should evaluate the operator for infection control, ability to communicate effectively, and "bedside" manner. Rotate these positions every hour to ensure that all students have an opportunity to serve in each role.

Worksheet #1

Record your findings from Critical Thinking Activity #5 on this worksheet. Check off the boxes as you work to identify each instrument.

	Instrument 1	Instrument 2	Instrument 3	Instrument 4	Instrument 5	Instrument 6
Single ended						
Double ended						
Paired ends						
Shank						
Short						
Long						
Straight						
Angled						
Working end						
Parallel cutting edges						
Convergent cutting edges						
One cutting edge is higher						
Single cutting edge						
Lateral sides from a point						
Lateral sides converge to a rounded toe						
Lateral sides contain calibrated markings						

Instrument Identification

Chisel						
Hoe						
Sickle						
Universal curet						
Area-specific curet						
Probe						
Explorer						

Chapter **9** **Instrument Design and Principles of Instrumentation**

DO I have all the answers?

Review Questions

Check your answers against the Answer Key at the back of this Study Guide to assess what you have learned.

1. One of the instruments on the tray in the first Critical Thinking Activity has a working end with two straight cutting edges that join to form a point. This instrument is most likely which one of the following?
   a. Curet
   b. Sickle
   c. Hoe
   d. File
   e. Explorer

2. Another instrument on the tray has two straight cutting edges that join to form a rounded toe. This instrument is most likely which one of the following?
   a. Curet
   b. Sickle
   c. Hoe
   d. File
   e. Explorer

3. Instruments with multiple straight cutting edges parallel to one another are most likely called which one of the following?
   a. Curets
   b. Sickles
   c. Hoes
   d. Files
   e. Explorers

4. The advantages of the use of instruments with wide hollow handles include which one of the following?
   a. Improves tactile sensitivity
   b. Prevents finger fatigue
   c. Improves instrument control
   d. All of the above
   e. None of the above

5. A variation in the thickness of the instrument shank has an effect on the amount of calculus that can be removed. Thin flexible shanks remove fine calculus deposits, whereas thicker, more rigid shanks remove moderate-to-heavy calculus deposits.
   a. The statement is correct, but the reason is not.
   b. The statement is incorrect, but the reason is correct.
   c. Both statement and reason are correct.
   d. Both statement and reason are incorrect.

6. In a proper modified pen grasp, which one of the following is correct?
   a. Index finger, middle finger, and thumb create a tripod on the instrument handle.
   b. Pads of index finger and thumb are opposite each other on the handle, whereas the middle finger rests on the shank.
   c. Middle finger area adjacent to the shank rests on the ring finger.
   d. Tip of the ring finger serves as the fulcrum.
   e. All of the above are correct.

7. An intraoral fulcrum provides which one of the following functions?
   a. Prevents operator fatigue
   b. Prevents injury to the patient
   c. Enables hand and instrument to move as a unit
   d. All of the above
   e. None of the above

8. In which of the following ways is proper adaptation of the instrument's working end to the tooth surface maintained during activation?
   a. By rotating the instrument between the index finger and thumb
   b. By squeezing the instrument between the index finger and thumb
   c. By pushing down on the fulcrum finger
   d. By moving the instrument handle away from the tooth
   e. None of the above

9. The angle formed by the face of the working end of the instrument to the tooth surface to remove calculus should be which one of the following?
   a. Less than 45 degrees
   b. Greater than 90 degrees
   c. Less than 90 degrees
   d. Greater than 45 degrees
   e. Both *c* and *d*

10. Which one of the following best describes the proper scaling stroke?
    a. Short and firm
    b. Overlapping
    c. Vertical or oblique
    d. Engages edge of deposit
    e. All of the above

11. The use of an ultrasonic scaler removes which one of the following?
    a. Supragingival calculus
    b. Subgingival calculus
    c. Plaque
    d. *a* only
    e. *a*, *b*, and *c*

WHERE do I go for more information or support?

evolve

For suggested web sites and agencies, additional readings and resources, and more chapter-specific information, please consult your Evolve Student Resources. Because of the ever-changing nature of the Internet, please keep in mind that web sites listed and their content may change.

CD-ROM

Reference files: As you work through the CD-ROM exercises, you should be able to print reference files and add them to your class materials. No specific reference files apply to this chapter.

HOW can I keep track of my progress toward competence?

As an ongoing picture of progress, record and monitor clinical experiences relating to Chapter 9 content in your Portfolio.

Self-Reflection

On a regular basis, review these experiences (with a faculty member). Identify strengths, weaknesses (not just numbers), and changes that you would incorporate into your clinical care plan now that you have had these experiences.

10 Instrument Sharpening

WHY do I need to know about Instrument Sharpening?

Instrument sharpening techniques, critical to successful instrumentation, are often learned early in the dental hygiene curriculum. Unfortunately, many dental hygiene students hold the misconception that they will never have to sharpen an instrument in private practice! Eventually, every dental hygienist realizes that maintaining sharp instruments will ultimately make hand-scaling procedures more effective and efficient. In 1908, G.V. Black recognized the effectiveness of sharp instruments; his thoughts are reinforced daily in dental hygiene practice. Simply stated, periodontal debridement cannot be accomplished with dull instruments. Learning proper sharpening techniques early and developing good, consistent sharpening procedures will keep instruments sharp and ready for the procedures to be performed.

WHAT will I be able to do with this knowledge?

1. Value the need for sharp instruments and demonstrate sharpening as indicated by the criteria in this chapter.
2. Compare and contrast the various types of sharpening methods and equipment.
3. Compare and contrast the variety of handheld stones available for sharpening.
4. Explain the rationale in selecting particular sharpening stones.
5. Select an appropriate sharpening method for instrument design, and explain the rationale for the selection.
6. Debate the pros and cons of the sharpening techniques that remove metal from the lateral sides of the working end or from the face of the blade.
7. Explain the rationale used to learn the stationary instrument–moving stone technique over the moving instrument–stationary stone technique.
8. Explain the care and maintenance of all varieties of sharpening stones.
9. Demonstrate the steps used to sharpen each of the following instruments: sickles with flame-shaped cutting edges, sickles with straight cutting edges, Gracey curets, universal curets, hoe scalers, disk scalers, files, and explorers.

HOW do I prepare myself to transfer this knowledge to patient care?

Go to Chapter 10 content on your CD-ROM or search for "Instrument Sharpening."

CD Exercises

- *10-1: Manual Sharpening Methods: Straight Sickle Scaler—Video:* Identify appropriate grasp, stone position, and sharpening stroke for a straight scaler.
- *10-2: Manual Sharpening Methods: Curved Sickle Scaler—Video:* Identify appropriate grasp, stone position, and sharpening stroke for a curved scaler.
- *10-3: Manual Sharpening Methods: Universal Curet—Video:* Identify appropriate grasp, stone position, and stroke of sharpening for a universal curet.
- *10-4: Manual Sharpening Methods: Area-Specific Curet—Video:* Identify appropriate grasp, stone position, and stroke of sharpening for an area-specific curet.
- *10-5: Common Technique Errors: Identifying Error—Video:* Identify the type of sharpening error that resulted in the instruments shown.

Textbook

Review Case Study 10-1, Disadvantages of Using a Dull Instrument, and the case applications.

For important concepts and application of knowledge, the following text elements may be especially helpful for clinical transfer and may be used as a clinical resource:

- Table 10-1
- Boxes 10-1 through 10-6
- Figures 10-2, 10-6, 10-8 through 10-29

HOW do I perform these skills?

evolve

A printable version of this checklist is available on your Evolve Student Resources.

To sharpen an instrument correctly, I will:

☐ Lubricate the stone based on manufacturer's suggestions.

☐ Grasp the instrument to be sharpened in a palm grasp or modified pen grasp with the nondominant hand placed against the countertop.

- Rest the hand holding the instrument on the table-top and the instrument handle against the edge of the countertop.
- Point the toe of the instrument toward the clinician and the face of the blade parallel to the floor.
- Hold the stone in my dominant hand.
- Position the stone on the lateral side of the instrument, near the heel of the working end at a 90-degree angle to the face of the blade.
- Begin the sharpening motion on a downstroke, moving the stone down and up while maintaining the 100- to 110-degree angulation.
- Stop the sharpening procedure on a downstroke to reduce the chance of creating a wire edge.
- Reposition the stone on the lateral side of the opposite cutting edge of the instrument near the heel at a 90-degree angle.
- Wipe the sludge from the instrument.
- Test the instrument.
- Sharpen the opposite cutting edge using steps as stated previously.
- Remove any wire edges.

HOW can I more effectively use this knowledge?

Critical Thinking Activities

Use the following worksheet to complete activity #1.

1. Obtain a variety of used instruments. Examine the working end of each instrument for design and shape. Determine whether the shape has been altered from sharpening in any way. If it has, then identify sharpening errors that could have caused the current shape.
2. View extremely dull instruments under a high-intensity lamp. Observe the shiny line along the cutting edge. Compare a brand new instrument with the dull instrument under a high-intensity lamp. What differences can you detect?
3. Sharpen an extremely dull instrument. Before removing the sludge, observe the cutting edge under a high-intensity lamp with a magnifying glass. Look for a wire edge or a layer of sludge or both.
4. Coat the roots of sterilized extracted teeth with nail polish and corn meal. When the coating has dried, scale the root surfaces with dull instruments. Observe the pressure and difficulty during attempts to remove the deposits with dull instruments. Now, sharpen the dull instruments and repeat the process. Observe the ease of deposit removal.
5. Observe a clinician in private practice during an instrumentation procedure. Ask the clinician's opinion on sharpening procedures, and observe the technique. What observations can you make? Is the technique the same as what you have been taught? How does it differ? What steps did the clinician follow when sharpening during the appointment? When are instruments sharpened in that practice?

Worksheet #1

Record your findings from Critical Thinking Activity #1 on this worksheet. Using the following set of error codes, evaluate sharpened instruments to identify the error. Place the error number in the corresponding column and identify what may have caused the sharpening error.

Error Code

1 = Toe has become pointed.
2 = Toe has become rounded.
3 = Two cutting edges are visible.
4 = Cutting edges have become parallel.
5 = Cutting edges are no longer parallel.
6 = Blade has been shortened.

Image Number	Error Code	Cause of Error
1		
2		
3		
4		
5		
6		
7		
8		
9		
10		

Review Questions

Check your answers against the Answer Key at the back of this Study Guide to assess what you have learned.
Question 1 refers to Case Study 10-1.

1. Which one of the following can occur through the use of dull instruments for debridement?
   a. Operator can lose tactile sensitivity for calculus detection.
   b. Calculus can be burnished into the root surface during debridement.
   c. Instrument can slip during debridement, resulting in injury to the patient.
   d. Operator may have to increase pressure to the instrument for calculus removal.
   e. All of the above can occur.

2. Which one of the following procedures would be ideal to maintain desirable instrument sharpness throughout the debridement process?
   a. Sharpen instruments at the beginning of each day.
   b. Keep sterile sharpening equipment available for all procedures.
   c. Sharpen instruments before placing them in the autoclave.
   d. Use a magnifying glass while sharpening.

3. When the sharpening stone is correctly applied to a sickle or curet just before activation, which one of the following describes the angle formed by the stone to the face of the blade?
   a. 70 to 80 degrees
   b. 60 to 80 degrees
   c. 45 to 90 degrees
   d. 100 to 110 degrees

4. Which one of the following procedures is appropriate to sharpen a flame-shaped sickle scaler?
   a. Keep the stone in constant contact with the entire length of the cutting edge of the instrument.
   b. Hold the instrument in a pen grasp.
   c. Place the stone at the heel of the instrument, and follow the contour of the cutting edge to the tip.
   d. Use long strokes with heavy pressure on the downstroke.

5. Which visible cue can the clinician use to assume the cutting edge of the instrument is sharp?
   a. Clinician may observe the wire edge on the blade.
   b. Edge will reflect light and will appear bright and shiny.
   c. Edge will not reflect light and will appear as a dull line.
   d. Edge will have a layer of sludge.

6. Which one of the following is the initial placement of the instrument against the sharpening stone before the sharpening procedure is initiated?
   a. 60 degrees
   b. 90 degrees
   c. 100 degrees
   d. 110 degrees

7. When the hoe is sharpened, which one of the following is *true?*
   a. Entire cutting edge is against the stone.
   b. Handle is approximately 70 degrees from the stone.
   c. Instrument is held in a modified pen grasp with a finger rest on the stone.
   d. Beveled toe is placed flat on the stone.
   e. All of the above are true.

8. When the universal curet is sharpened, which one of the following is *true?*
   a. Stone should contact the entire cutting edge from heel to toe.
   b. Instrument is used in a pen grasp.
   c. Stone is placed at the heel of the instrument and follows the contour of the cutting edge to the toe.
   d. Long strokes with heavy pressure are used.

9. To round the toe of an area-specific curet, which one of the following techniques is *not* correct?
   a. Round from both cutting edges of the same working end.
   b. Round from one cutting edge of the working end.
   c. Increase stone-to-face angle by 15 to 25 degrees.
   d. Round the toe every fourth or fifth time the instrument is sharpened.

10. When sharpening an area-specific curet, the clinician should perform which one of the following?
    a. Hold the instrument in a pen grasp.
    b. Place the stone at the heel of the instrument, and follow the contour of the cutting edge to the toe.
    c. Make sure the stone is in contact with the entire cutting edge of the instrument from heel to toe.
    d. Use long strokes with heavy pressure.

WHERE do I go for more information or support?

For suggested web sites and agencies, additional readings and resources, and more chapter-specific information, please consult your Evolve Student Resources. Because of the ever-changing nature of the Internet, please keep in mind that web sites listed and their content may change.

CD-ROM

Reference files: As you work through the CD-ROM exercises, you should be able to print reference files and add them to your class materials. No specific reference files apply to this chapter.

HOW can I keep track of my progress toward competence?

As an ongoing picture of progress, record and monitor clinical experiences relating to Chapter 10 content in your Portfolio.

Self-Reflection

On a regular basis, review these experiences (with a faculty member). Identify strengths, weaknesses (not just numbers), and changes that you would incorporate into your clinical care plan now that you have had these experiences.

11 Life Stages

WHY do I need to know about Life Stages?

Each patient has age-dependent needs that a clinician should take into account in assessment, treatment, and oral health instruction. These age-dependent variables can take on many forms, from physical to psychologic to physiologic, as well as combinations of all three forms. The clinician must be aware and alert to the implications these variables have on treatment and treatment outcomes.

WHAT will I be able to do with this knowledge?

1. Institute anticipatory guidance principles of health outcomes with patients in each life stage.
2. Identify specific patient needs, as identified for each life stage.
3. Develop patient relationships based on the knowledge of issues relative to each life stage of patients.
4. Understand the relationship between the biological and psychosocial aspects of patient care.
5. Explain the menstrual cycle process.
6. Discuss the relationship of hormonal changes to systemic and oral health.
7. Apply issues specific to the various life stages to the development of preventive and therapeutic interventions.

HOW do I prepare myself to transfer this knowledge to patient care?

Go to Chapter 11 content on your CD-ROM or search for "Life Stages."

CD Exercises

- *11-1: Life Stages—All Patients :* Determine appropriate life stage, anatomical and dental development, and physiologic development and anticipatory guidance for each representative age group (represented on all patient cases on CD-ROM).
- *11-2 to 11-7:* Select specific anticipatory guidance topics based on patient needs (must see all records).

- *Additional Exercise:* Select the following patients from the patient menu on the CD-ROM. Review their charts to design appointment parameters using the anticipatory guidance approach appropriate for each patient's age. *Use the following worksheets to complete your activities.*
  - Worksheet #1: Terrence Zellar
  - Worksheet #2: Subra Mani
  - Worksheet #3: Adolfo Santana
  - Worksheet #4: Maria Bjork
  - Worksheet #5: Ann Cronin
  - Worksheet #6: Elena Guri

Textbook

Review Case Study 11-1, Appreciating Life Stage Changes to Build Rapport and Guide Treatment, and the case applications.

For important concepts and application of knowledge, the following text elements may be especially helpful for clinical transfer and may be used as a clinical resource:
- Tables 11-1 through 11-5
- Figures 11-1, 11-3, 11-6, 11-9, and 11-11

HOW can I more effectively use this knowledge?

Critical Thinking Activities

1. Develop a training activity program to take into a nursing home to present to the residents. Keep in mind what physical, psychologic, and medical issues they may be experiencing as you develop your program.
2. Develop a series of educational brochures, one for each life stage, and submit them to various organizations or corporations to seek support for broad distribution, especially to underserved populations.
3. Think of interactive educational activities for preschool children that would provide them useful yet entertaining and engaging oral health education.
4. Investigate the various cultural differences that may accompany each life stage, and develop a short educational module for one or more of them. Try to obtain

funding for distribution to the particular group you have chosen to develop your module around.

5. Investigate the various systemic diseases that are influenced by oral health disease, and develop a short article that can be released to the local media.

6. Compile a list of common hormone replacement medications and oral contraceptives, and review drug information sheets for oral effects.

7. Interview obstetric and gynecologic physicians and nurses regarding patient education on oral effects of hormonal imbalances.

8. Prepare a dental health education program for a prenatal class related to hormonal imbalances and effects on the oral cavity during pregnancy.

Worksheet #1

Use the following worksheets to complete information for the designated patients on your CD-ROM.

Patient Name: Terrence Zellar

Age

_____

Anatomical concerns

_____

_____

Pathologic concerns

_____

_____

Physiologic concerns

_____

_____

Topics for discussion

_____

_____

Actual clinical findings

_____

_____

Worksheet #2

Patient Name: Subra Mani

Age

_____

Anatomical concerns

_____

_____

Pathologic concerns

_____

_____

Physiologic concerns

_____

_____

Topics for discussion

_____

_____

Actual clinical findings

_____

_____

Worksheet #3

Patient Name: Adolfo Santana

Age

_____

Anatomical concerns

_____

_____

Pathologic concerns

_____

_____

Physiologic concerns

_____

_____

Topics for discussion

_____

_____

Actual clinical findings

_____

_____

Worksheet #4

Patient Name: Maria Bjork

Age

_____

Anatomical concerns

_____

_____

Pathologic concerns

_____

_____

Physiologic concerns

_____

_____

Topics for discussion

_____

_____

Actual clinical findings

_____

_____

Worksheet #5

Patient Name: Ann Cronin

Age _____

Anatomical concerns _____

_____

Pathologic concerns _____

_____

Physiologic concerns _____

_____

Topics for discussion _____

_____

Actual clinical findings _____

_____

Worksheet #6

Patient Name: Elena Guri

Age _____

Anatomical concerns _____

_____

Pathologic concerns _____

_____

Physiologic concerns _____

_____

Topics for discussion _____

_____

Actual clinical findings _____

_____

DO I have all the answers?

Review Questions

Check your answers against the Answer Key at the back of this Study Guide to assess what you have learned. Questions 1 and 9 refer to Case Study 11-1.

1. In which of the following statements is anticipatory guidance used appropriately with Georgette, the 15-year-old patient introduced in this chapter?
   a. "I see that you are beginning to accumulate a lot of plaque around the gums. It will be best if you can start to pay more attention to that and remove it on a daily basis."
   b. "You need to floss your teeth more often! You already have a significant amount of gingival bleeding."
   c. "Your teeth are so beautiful. To keep them looking that way you should floss them every day, especially because you are going into a period of development during which you will experience a significant change in your hormones. Amazingly, that increase in hormones can lead to periodontal disease if you are not aware of how to prevent it."
   d. "I know that your parents are concerned about the health of your teeth and have invested a lot of time and expense so that you can have a healthy mouth. You should pay more attention to how you take care of them so that you will not disappoint your parents."
2. The method of assessment and treatment planning presented in this chapter can best be described as which of the following?
   a. Medical model
   b. Biopsychosocial model
   c. Prevention model
   d. None of the above
3. Which aspects of someone's life could be affected by serious and visible dental caries?
   a. Perception of self
   b. Perceived locus of control
   c. Amount of social interaction
   d. All of the above
4. To effectively use anticipatory guidance in your work with your patients, which of the following is (are) important?
   a. Anticipation of patient needs
   b. Understanding of the patients' particular life circumstances
   c. Knowledge of life stages and the general health-related events that accompany those stages
   d. All of the above
5. The condition known as *early childhood caries (ECC)* is *not* initiated with which of the following when the infant is put to bed?
   a. Giving an infant a bottle with fluoridated water
   b. Giving an infant a bottle with fortified milk
   c. Giving an infant a bottle with a fruit drink
   d. Giving an infant a bottle with soda pop

6. The nonnutritive sucking habit does not provide which of the following benefits?
   a. Calming effect
   b. Self-regulation
   c. Control of emotions
   d. Improved coordination
7. The outcome faced by children who experience a high level of oral disease includes which of the following?
   a. Persistent dental pain
   b. Inability to eat comfortably
   c. Embarrassment with peers
   d. Potential for poor nutrition
   e. All of the above
8. Which of the following can affect tooth development in the fetus?
   a. Alcohol consumption
   b. Poor posture
   c. Illegal drug use
   d. Poor nutrition
   e. *a, c,* and *d*
9. All of the following behaviors can result in successful therapy with adolescent patients, such as Georgette from Case Study 11-1. Which one is the *exception?*
   a. Listening to their concerns
   b. Demanding that they change their oral care habits
   c. Showing an interest in who they are outside of the dental office
   d. Complimenting them on some aspect of their oral health care regimen
10. Which of the following female sex hormones is responsible for changes in the endometrium during the second half of the menstrual cycle?
    a. Estrogen
    b. Progesterone
11. Progesterone affects the health of gingival tissues in which of the following ways?
    a. Dilation of capillaries
    b. Decrease in keratinization
    c. Increase in vascular permeability
    d. Alterations in collagen production
12. Which of the following is characterized by enlarged, bluish-red, and bulbous tissue?
    a. Puberty gingivitis
    b. Pregnancy gingivitis
    c. Gingivitis associated with oral contraceptive use
    d. Menopausal gingivostomatitis
13. Oral surgery procedures should be scheduled during which days of the oral contraceptive cycle?
    a. Days 7 to 12
    b. Days 13 to 18
    c. Days 19 to 22
    d. Days 23 to 28

WHERE do I go for more information or support?

evolve

For suggested web sites and agencies, additional readings and resources, and more chapter-specific information, please consult your Evolve Student Resources. Because of the ever-changing nature of the Internet, please keep in mind that web sites listed and their content may change.

💿 CD-ROM

Reference files: As you work through the CD-ROM exercises, you should be able to print reference files and add them to your class materials. This information includes patient-specific assessment forms that may be related to the activities in Chapter 11.

HOW can I keep track of my progress toward competence?

As an ongoing picture of progress, record and monitor clinical experiences relating to Chapter 11 content in your Portfolio.

Self-Reflection

On a regular basis, review these experiences (with a faculty member). Identify strengths, weaknesses (not just numbers), and changes that you would incorporate into your clinical care plan now that you have had these experiences.

12 Comprehensive Health History

WHY do I need to know about Comprehensive Health History?

The dental hygienist must be aware of the implications of systemic diseases and illness to prevent harm to patients and to provide safe and effective care. Studying the diseases associated with each organ system, knowing signs, and recognizing symptoms will aid in developing a professional approach to oral health care. Obtaining, accurately recording, and evaluating a comprehensive health history will help ensure successful treatment outcomes.

WHAT will I be able to do with this knowledge?

1. Identify the essential components of a comprehensive patient health history.
2. List the parts of each component of the health history.
3. Recognize the importance of each component of the health history to the acquisition of an accurate health database.
4. Analyze verbal and written patient responses to the health questionnaire to anticipate and initiate the needed modifications in the treatment plan.
5. Analyze verbal and written patient responses to the health questionnaire to recognize when a medical or dental consultation is warranted.

HOW do I prepare myself to transfer this knowledge to patient care?

 Go to Chapter 12 content on your CD-ROM or search for "Health History."

CD Exercises

■ *12-1 to 12-3: Process of Obtaining the Health History:* Identify the next question concerning health history inquiry for patients Ann Cronin, Eva Bjork, and Adolfo Santana.

Textbook

Review Case Study 12-1, Significance of a Thorough Health History, and the case applications. Take the time to answer the case application questions regarding Case Study 12-1 at the beginning of the chapter.

HOW do I perform these skills?

evolve

A printable version of this checklist is available on your Evolve Student Resources.
To provide a comprehensive health and dental history review, I will:
□ Prevent or minimize interference with the patient's medical status when planning dental treatment.
□ Recognize medical conditions and be able to monitor a patient's physical status to ensure that his or her medical condition is stable.
□ Be aware of the patient's medications, the drug actions, and the potential drug interactions.
□ Document findings in chart, as appropriate.

HOW can I more effectively use this knowledge?

Critical Thinking Activities

Use the following worksheets to complete activity #3.
1. The dental hygienist often refers to a medical reference textbook. In the index area in the back of *The Merck Manual* (Merck & Co. Available on the Internet: http://www.merck.com/mrkshared/mmanual/home.jsp Accessed Sept 2006.), become familiar with looking up specific diseases and locating diseases in the main text. For example, look up *sickle cell anemia, bradycardia, cataracts,* and *eclampsia.*
2. Refer to a drug reference textbook (e.g., *Mosby's Dental Drug Reference* [Mosby]). In the index in the back of the reference book, become familiar with looking up specific medications and locating medications in the main text area. Focus on the actions and pharmacodynamics, the route and dose, the contraindications and precautions, the adverse effects and side effects, and the relationship to dental hygiene care.
3. Using Worksheet #1:
   a. Review the medications of the CD-ROM patients indicated on the following worksheets. Identify medications each patient is taking, and look up each medication in a drug reference manual.

b. Look up the diseases or disorders listed on the medical history in a medical reference manual.
c. Assess the relationship between the patient's medication or medications and the identified medical problems.
4. Review three to five health histories of clinic patients in each of the following age ranges and determine where they fall in the grid for disease incidence and death, as presented in this chapter:
a. 1 to 19 years (men and women)
b. 20 to 39 years (men and women)
c. 40 to 59 years (men and women)
d. 60 to 79 years (men and women)
e. 80 years and older (men and women)
   What conclusions can you draw based on your observations? Might any personal habits have changed their health profiles, such as smoking or exercise?

5. Review your clinic medical or dental history forms. Are there any additions or deletions you would make based on this chapter?
6. Role-play with a peer, explaining the importance of a thorough medical and dental history. The "patient" should be unwilling to complete such a "long" form and should want to know why all this "stuff" is necessary. "After all," the patient may say, "I am just having my teeth cleaned."
7. Identify which portions of the organ systems review, when answered positively, place a patient at increased risk for dental disease.
8. Identify which portions of the dental history review, when answered positively, place a patient at increased risk for systemic disease.

Worksheet #1

Read the directions for Critical Thinking Activity #3. Review the medical histories on a patient in your clinic and for one or more of the following CD-ROM patients: Ann Cronin, William Johnston, George Burkett, and Elena Guri.

Record the indicated uses, side effects, adverse reactions, contraindications, and precautions for each medication each patient is taking. Then record any dental considerations associated with the medication. One worksheet will be required for each drug reviewed.

Patient Name _____

Medication _____

_____

_____

Uses _____

_____

_____

Side effects _____

_____

_____

Adverse reactions _____

_____

_____

_____

Contraindications _____

_____

_____

Precautions _____

_____

_____

Dental considerations _____

_____

_____

Continued
59

Patient Name _____

Medication _____

_____

_____

Uses _____

_____

_____

Side effects _____

_____

_____

Adverse reactions _____

_____

_____

Contraindications _____

_____

_____

Precautions _____

_____

_____

Dental considerations _____

_____

_____

Chapter **12** **Comprehensive Health History**

Worksheet #1—cont'd

Patient Name _____

Medication _____

_____

_____

Uses _____

_____

_____

Side effects _____

_____

_____

Adverse reactions _____

_____

_____

Contraindications _____

_____

_____

Precautions _____

_____

_____

Dental considerations _____

_____

_____

Continued

61

Worksheet #1—cont'd

Patient Name _____

Medication _____

_____

_____

Uses _____

_____

_____

Side effects _____

_____

_____

Adverse reactions _____

_____

_____

Contraindications _____

_____

_____

Precautions _____

_____

_____

Dental considerations _____

_____

_____

Chapter **12   Comprehensive Health History**

Worksheet #1—cont'd

Patient Name _____

Medication _____

_____

_____

Uses _____

_____

_____

Side effects _____

_____

Adverse reactions _____

_____

_____

Contraindications _____

_____

_____

Precautions _____

_____

_____

Dental considerations _____

_____

_____

DO I have all the answers?

Review Questions

Check your answers against the Answer Key at the back of this Study Guide to assess what you have learned.

1. The essential elements of a health history include all *except* which of the following?
   a. Full-mouth radiographic survey
   b. Vital signs
   c. Patient identification
   d. History of present oral condition (chief complaint)
   e. Social history

2. The history of a patient's present oral condition would include which of the following examples?
   a. Glucotrol by mouth for diabetes
   b. Blood pressure of 180/98 mm Hg
   c. Dull, constant pain in upper right molar
   d. 40-year history of cigarette smoking

3. All of the following are components of the social history *except one*. Which component is the exception?
   a. Alcohol use
   b. Emotional status
   c. Occupation
   d. Age
   e. Level of education

4. The American Heart Association recommends that certain dental patients receive antimicrobial premedications before a dental prophylaxis. For which of the following conditions would premedication be recommended?
   a. History of rheumatic fever (RF)
   b. Functional heart murmur (HM)
   c. Prosthetic aortic valve
   d. Myocardial infarction (MI) 3 years ago

5. During the past 10 years, the incidence of tuberculosis (TB) has increased. Which of the following would indicate active (infectious) TB in a dental patient?
   a. Positive purified protein derivative (PPD) test
   b. Negative PPD test
   c. History of taking isoniazid for 6 months
   d. Positive sputum
   e. Negative chest radiograph

6. Common oral findings in the patient with diabetes include all *except* which of the following?
   a. Xerostomia
   b. Candidiasis
   c. Progressive periodontal disease
   d. Caries
   e. Fluorosis

WHERE do I go for more information or support?

evolve

For suggested web sites and agencies, additional readings and resources, and more chapter-specific information, please consult your Evolve Student Resources. Because of the ever-changing nature of the Internet, please keep in mind that web sites listed and their content may change.

CD-ROM

Reference files: As you work through the CD-ROM exercises, you should be able to print reference files and add them to your class materials. No specific reference files apply to this chapter.

HOW can I keep track of my progress toward competence?

As an ongoing picture of progress, record and monitor clinical experiences relating to Chapter 12 content in your Portfolio.

Self-Reflection

On a regular basis, review these experiences (with a faculty member). Identify strengths, weaknesses (not just numbers), and changes that you would incorporate into your clinical care plan now that you have had these experiences.

13 Drug-Induced Adverse Oral Events

WHY do I need to know about Drug-Induced Adverse Oral Events?

Dental hygienists treat many patients who are taking medications. Invariably, they encounter issues related to drugs and their use, including drug indications, adverse events, drug interactions, and factors affecting adherence. Additionally, managing oral side effects of medications remains an ongoing challenge for dental hygienists. The ability to evaluate these issues, accurately assess the patient's status, and plan for medication-related prevention and treatment interventions is an essential part of the dental hygiene process of care.

WHAT will I be able to do with this knowledge?

1. Conduct a thorough pharmacologic history review to determine whether the patient's medication use has the potential to cause adverse oral events.
2. Assess the patient's medication list to identify those medications associated with adverse oral side effects.
3. Identify strategies used to prevent or treat medication-induced adverse oral events.
4. Confidently discuss the relationship of the patient's chief complaint, oral presentation, and medications with the patient, the patient's physician, and the dentist.

HOW do I prepare myself to transfer this knowledge to patient care?

 Go to Chapter 13 content on your CD-ROM or search for "Medications" or "Side Effects."

CD Exercises

- *13-1: Oral Manifestations of Common Medications:* Select common oral manifestations of 23 medication categories to learn how to identify their clinical signs. Write this information to a reference file.
- *13-2 to 13-4: Oral Manifestations of Common Medications:* Determine possible oral effects of medications taken in the following patients: Ann Cronin, William Johnston, and Elena Guri.

Textbook

Review Case Study 13-1, Erythema Multiforme, and the case application.

HOW do I perform these skills?

evolve

A printable version of this checklist is available on your Evolve Student Resources.
To assess the drug-induced adverse oral event accurately, I will:

- ☐ Identify the patient's chief oral complaint as it relates to his or her medications.
- ☐ Develop a differential diagnosis of the patient's chief complaint to include the medication as an etiologic factor.
- ☐ Evaluate oral conditions that vary from normal and determine a drug-induced adverse oral event from the medications reported taken by the patient.
- ☐ Confidently discuss the relationship between the patient's chief complaint and medications with the patient's physician and dentist.
- ☐ Document findings and discussion in chart.

HOW can I more effectively use this knowledge?

Critical Thinking Activities

Use the following worksheet to complete activity #2.

1. Prepare a handout for patients' use describing the oral side effects of the following drugs and steps they can take to reduce the side effects:
   - Antidepressants
   - Phenytoin
   - Nifedipine
2. Using the CD-ROM patients indicated on Worksheet #1, review the medication history and correlate the history to the dental charting and patient prescriptions. Can you find any oral symptoms in the record that could be related to the medication listing?
3. You are completing a health history on an older patient (age 75) with an extensive medication history. He

wants to know why you need to know "all that stuff." How would you reply?

4. Survey a family member to identify all medications the person is taking. Using a drug reference book, list the potential oral adverse effects of the medications. Inquire as to whether the person currently experiences any of the effects.

5. Role-play discussions with healthcare providers (i.e., dentists, physicians) concerning oral manifestations based on the patient's intake of certain medications.

6. Develop a ready reference for management of specific clinical oral lesions based on specific medications.

Worksheet #1

Using the form provided, complete Critical Thinking Activity #2 and determine oral side effects from the medications being taken by some of the patients on the CD-ROM. Indicate measures to reduce side effect when applicable.

Patient Name	Medication History	Potential Oral Side Effect	Clinical Manifestation
Ann Cronin			
William Johnston			
Elena Guri			
George Burkett			

Chapter **13** **Drug-Induced Adverse Oral Events**

DO I have all the answers?

Review Questions

Check your answers against the Answer Key at the back of this Study Guide to assess what you have learned.

1. Which one of the following conditions produces the most common drug-related adverse oral event?
   a. Lichenoid drug reaction
   b. Candidiasis
   c. Dysgeusia
   d. Xerostomia

2. *Candida albicans* has strong pathogenicity. It works with local or systemic factors to produce a diseased state.
   a. Both statements are true.
   b. Both statements are false.
   c. The first statement is true; the second statement is false.
   d. The first statement is false; the second statement is true.

3. Treatment of candidiasis includes topical and systemic antifungal therapy. Systemic antifungal therapy is more effective and the preferred treatment of choice.
   a. Both statements are true.
   b. Both statements are false.
   c. The first statement is true; the second statement is false.
   d. The first statement is false; the second statement is true.

4. A patient has ulcerative lesions of the oral mucosa and "iris" lesions of the skin. Medical history reveals a recent onset of sore throat and fever, which was treated with trimethoprim-sulfamethoxazole (TMP-SMZ). The patient reports that lesions were noted several days after use of this medication. Which one of the following conditions is the most likely diagnosis for this reaction?
   a. Lichenoid drug reaction
   b. Erythema multiforme (EM)
   c. Candidiasis
   d. Stevens-Johnson syndrome

5. Which one of the following diagnostic tests is most useful in determining a lichenoid drug reaction?
   a. Withdraw the medication
   b. Biopsy
   c. Indirect immunofluorescence
   d. Medical history

6. Mr. Smith has a lichenoid drug reaction. He reports taking the following medications: atorvastatin calcium (Lipitor), metformin hydrochloride (Glucophage), aspirin, multivitamins, glucosamine, and chondroitin sulfate. Which one of these medications would most likely cause a lichenoid drug reaction?
   a. Glucophage
   b. Lipitor
   c. Aspirin
   d. Chondroitin sulfate

7. Which one of the following medications are most thought to be associated with drug-induced gingival enlargement?
   a. Divalproex sodium (Depakote) and verapamil
   b. Phenytoin and nifedipine
   c. Phenytoin and verapamil
   d. Depakote and nifedipine

8. Which one of the following is most related to the pathogenesis of drug-induced gingival enlargement?
   a. Dose of specific medications
   b. Increased dental plaque
   c. Direct effects of cellular targets
   d. All of the above

9. Hairy tongue is a benign hyperkeratinization of which papillae of the tongue?
   a. Filiform
   b. Fungiform
   c. Circumvallate
   d. All of the above

10. When oral antihistamines are not successful in the treatment of angioedema, which one of the following is the next course of treatment to be administered?
    a. Intravenous (IV) corticosteroids
    b. Intramuscular (IM) antihistamines
    c. IV antihistamines
    d. IM epinephrine

WHERE do I go for more information or support?

evolve

For suggested web sites and agencies, additional readings and resources, and more chapter-specific information, please consult your Evolve Student Resources. Because of the ever-changing nature of the Internet, please keep in mind that web sites listed and their content may change.

CD-ROM

Reference files: The first exercise for Chapter 13 on the CD-ROM, *Oral Manifestations of Common Medications*, can be written to a reference file once you have completed it and printed it out to keep with your class materials.

HOW can I keep track of my progress toward competence?

As an ongoing picture of progress, record and monitor clinical experiences relating to Chapter 13 content in your Portfolio.

Self-Reflection

On a regular basis, review these experiences (with a faculty member). Identify strengths, weaknesses (not just numbers), and changes that you would incorporate into your clinical care plan now that you have had these experiences.

14 Physical and Extraoral Examination

WHY do I need to know about Physical and Extraoral Examination?

The dental hygienist is in an excellent position to assist in the diagnosis of pathologic systemic conditions. Recognition of normal anatomy and physiologic function, normal variations, and the early signs and symptoms of disease is important. These observations lead to a diagnosis and proper treatment.

WHAT will I be able to do with this knowledge?

1. Perform a thorough extraoral examination, identifying structures and abnormalities during the examination.
2. Take patients' vital signs according to techniques presented in the chapter.
3. Evaluate readings obtained when taking vital signs and identify whether precautions or consultations are needed before the performance of dental hygiene care.

HOW do I prepare myself to transfer this knowledge to patient care?

 Go to Chapter 14 content on your CD-ROM or search for "Extraoral Exam" or "Vital Signs."

CD Exercises

- *14-1: Palpation—Video:* Identify the type of palpation technique used from video observation.
- *14-2: Palpation—George Burkett:* Identify the type of palpation technique used on George Burkett.
- *14-3: Palpation:* Identify needed palpation technique for each specific site given.
- *14-4: Lymph Nodes—Reference File:* Build a chart of lymph nodes for the student reference file.
- *14-5: Lymph Nodes—George Burkett:* After watching a video clip, identify the lymph chain being palpated on George Burkett.
- *14-6: Salivary Glands—Reference File:* Build a chart of salivary glands for the student reference file.
- *14-7: Temperature—Reference File:* Build a chart for reference file of temperature readings.
- *14-8: Pulse—Reference File:* Build a chart for reference file of pulse readings.
- *14-9: Respiration—Reference File:* Build a chart for reference file of respiration readings.
- *14-10: Blood Pressure—Reference File:* Build a chart for reference file of blood pressure readings.
- *14-11 to 14-14: Blood Pressure:* Evaluate blood pressure in patients George Burkett, Maria Bjork, Subra Mani, and Adolfo Santana.

Textbook

Review Case Study 14-1, Examination Process, and the case applications.

HOW do I perform these skills?

evolve

A printable version of this checklist is available on your Evolve Student Resources.
To provide a thorough head and neck examination, I will:

- ☐ Evaluate and inspect each patient's body symmetry, posture, stature, and skin color and texture.
- ☐ Inspect eyes, ears, and nose for any abnormalities.
- ☐ Palpate laterally along the clavicles, pressing down into the supraclavicular triangle and the top of the clavicles using bidigital circular compression until the trapezius muscle is reached.
- ☐ Return to the sternum and palpate upward in the midline of the neck.
- ☐ Palpate the cricoid cartilage wand submental lymph nodes.
- ☐ Palpate under the chin and along the mandible.
- ☐ Palpate the anterior aspect of the sternocleidomastoid muscle.
- ☐ Palpate the carotid artery.
- ☐ Palpate the posterior aspect of the sternocleidomastoid muscle down to the insertion of the trapezius muscle, and then move posteriorly to the cervical spine.
- ☐ Bilaterally palpate up the cervical spine.
- ☐ Palpate anteriorly to the ears and the posterior auricular lymph nodes and the anteroauricular nodes.
- ☐ Palpate the temporalis muscle while the patient goes through mandibular excursions.

- ☐ Palpate masseter muscles, parotid gland, and facial lymph nodes.
- ☐ Document findings and procedure in chart.

HOW can I more effectively use this knowledge?

Critical Thinking Activities

Use the following worksheets to complete activities #1, #2, #3, #4, and #5.

1. Using Worksheet #1, take your blood pressure before and after a laboratory examination and note which number increased. Why do you think this number increased?
2. Using Worksheet #1, take your blood pressure and then drink 16 oz of water. Wait 20 minutes without urinating, retake your blood pressure, and compare the readings. Explain the difference noted in the readings.
3. Select records for patients Ann Cronin, George Burkett, Subra Mani, William Johnston, and Elena Guri from the CD-ROM. Record vital signs on Worksheet #2. Identify whether these are within normal ranges. Review the medical history and correlate your findings with the vital signs.
4. Evaluate the temporomandibular joint (TMJ) of a minimum of six classmates, family members, or others. Record your findings on Worksheet #3, identifying the number of individuals who had a problem with the TMJ based on your examination. Compare this with the individual's subjective appraisal of problems with this joint.
5. Using Worksheet #4, take a photograph of your face and the faces of a few classmates. Make sure the eyes are wide open. Draw a line through the midsagittal plane. Draw another line through the pupils. Assess for symmetry.
6. Investigate available blood pressure devices that can be discussed with patients, the value of these devices, their limitations, and basic operating procedure.

Worksheet #1

Use this worksheet with Critical Thinking Activity #1. Select three examination dates. Have a classmate take your blood pressure 20 minutes before the examination, and then 20 minutes after the examination.

Blood Pressure Reading

Date	Before Examination	After Examination
_____	___/___ mm Hg	___/___ mm Hg
_____	___/___ mm Hg	___/___ mm Hg
_____	___/___ mm Hg	___/___ mm Hg

Which reading increased (systolic or diastolic)? _____

What physiologic response can explain the increase? _____

Have a classmate take your blood pressure (resting rate), then drink 16 oz of water. After 20 minutes without urinating, have your blood pressure retaken. (See also Critical Thinking Activity #2.)

Blood Pressure Reading

Date	Resting:	After water ingestion:
_____	___/___ mm Hg	___/___ mm Hg

Which reading increased (systolic or diastolic)? _____

What physiologic response can explain the increase? _____

Chapter **14** **Physical and Extraoral Examination**

Worksheet #2

Use this worksheet with Critical Thinking Activity #3 to record your each patient's vital signs and other findings.

	Blood Pressure	Pulse	Within Normal Limits	Not Normal (in what way)	Medical History Correlation
Ann Cronin	___/___ mm Hg	___ bpm			
George Burkett	___/___ mm Hg	___ bpm			
Subra Mani	___/___ mm Hg	___ bpm			
William Johnston	___/___ mm Hg	___ bpm			
Elena Guri	___/___ mm Hg	___ bpm			

Chapter **14** **Physical and Extraoral Examination**

Worksheet #3

Use this worksheet with Critical Thinking Activity #4 to record your findings.

Temporomandibular Joint Examination

	Patient					
	1	2	3	4	5	6
Palpation Findings						
Tenderness						
Pain						
Auscultation						
Crepitus						
Cracking, popping						
Movements						
Smooth						
Deviation (left or right)						
Subluxation						
Patient Complaint						

Worksheet #4

Use this worksheet with Critical Thinking Activity #5 to record your findings.

Facial
Symmetry

Patient Observations

	1	2	3	4	5
Vertical symmetry					
Horizontal symmetry					

Review Questions

Check your answers against the Answer Key at the back of this Study Guide to assess what you have learned.

1. An examination of the lymph nodes of the head and neck region uses which one of the following examination techniques?
   a. Palpation
   b. Percussion
   c. Auscultation
   d. Probing

2. Examination of the TMJ uses which one of the following examination techniques?
   a. Probing and percussion
   b. Palpation and percussion
   c. Auscultation and palpation (listening)
   d. Auscultation and probing

3. A neoplastic lesion located on the ventrolateral surface of the tongue in the middle third of the tongue may result in an enlargement of which node?
   a. Submental
   b. Submandibular
   c. Jugulodigastric
   d. Mandibular (facial)

4. Periapical abscesses and severe, active periodontal disease may result in an enlargement of which lymph node?
   a. Submental
   b. Submandibular
   c. Jugulodigastric
   d. Mandibular (facial)

5. Which one of the following statements is *false?*
   a. The thyroid gland is located in the midline of the neck.
   b. A decrease in the size of the thyroid gland is consistent with a hypothyroid condition.
   c. Thyroid hormones regulate metabolic activities.
   d. An enlarged thyroid gland is a significant clinical finding.

6. Which one of the following statements is *false?*
   a. The parotid and submandibular salivary glands produce more than 90% of all saliva.
   b. The parotid gland located anterior to the ear secretes its saliva into the oral cavity via Stensen's duct.
   c. Salivary glands may become inflamed as a result of diabetes mellitus, lupus erythematosus (LE), and Sjögren's syndrome.
   d. The submandibular gland is located in the posterior mandible and thus cannot be palpated.

7. Which vital signs are elevated and increased or changed during an infection?
   a. Blood pressure, pulse, and respiration
   b. Temperature, heart rate, and respiration
   c. Blood pressure and temperature
   d. Respirations and blood pressure

8. Elective medical and dental procedures should not be performed when the patient's blood pressure is which one of the following?
   a. 140/90 mm Hg
   b. 180/110 mm Hg
   c. 140/80 mm Hg
   d. 130/90 mm Hg

9. Which one of the following statements is *false?*
   a. The dental healthcare provider can treat the hypertensive patient in the horizontal (reclined) position without any potential for an adverse occurrence.
   b. Infection is the leading cause for an elevated temperature.
   c. The dental healthcare provider may detect an undiagnosed hyperthyroid patient by assessing the pulse rate (extremely elevated, 110+).
   d. The hypertensive patient whose blood pressure is maintained in the normal range is not expected to develop end-organ damage.

10. The meniscus of the TMJ can be characterized by all of the following statements *except* one. Which one is the exception?
    a. The meniscus is fibrous and smooth.
    b. The posterior band of the meniscus cannot extend anterior to the condyle.
    c. The meniscus sits between the articular fossa and the convex articular eminence of the condyle.
    d. Tears or perforations of the meniscus can cause a grinding sound.

WHERE do I go for more information or support?

evolve

For suggested web sites and agencies, additional readings and resources, and more chapter-specific information, please consult your Evolve Student Resources. Because of the ever-changing nature of the Internet, please keep in mind that web sites listed and their content may change.

CD **CD-ROM**

Reference files: Several of the exercises for Chapter 14 should be written to a reference file once you have completed them:
- *14-4: Lymph Nodes*
- *14-6: Salivary Glands*
- *14-7: Temperature*
- *14-8: Pulse*
- *14-9: Respiration*
- *14-10: Blood Pressure*

Charts created for these exercises can be printed out to keep with your class materials.

HOW can I keep track of my progress toward competence?

As an ongoing picture of progress, record and monitor clinical experiences relating to Chapter 14 content in your Portfolio.

Self-Reflection

On a regular basis, review these experiences (with a faculty member). Identify strengths, weaknesses (not just numbers), and changes that you would incorporate into your clinical care plan now that you have had these experiences.

15 Intraoral Examination

WHY do I need to know about Intraoral Examination?

The dental hygienist must become familiar with the name, location, characteristics, and examination techniques of the intraoral anatomy. Only with this knowledge will the dental hygienist be able to provide appropriate patient care.

WHAT will I be able to do with this knowledge?

1. Identify the essential components of a comprehensive intraoral patient examination.
2. Recognize normal anatomical hard and soft tissue landmarks of the oral cavity.
3. Visually evaluate the integrity of the oral mucosa, noting any breaks that may exist and noting any irregularities in color or general appearance.
4. Determine tissue consistency (soft, firm, hard, nodular), tissue mobility (fixed, movable), and patient tenderness or discomfort using palpation and the sense of touch.
5. Assess anatomical bilateral symmetry for possible indications of underlying pathologic conditions.
6. Appropriately document both normal and abnormal findings.

HOW do I prepare myself to transfer this knowledge to patient care?

 Go to Chapter 15 content on your CD-ROM or search for "Intraoral Exam" or "Oral Anatomy."

CD Exercises

- *15-1: Intraoral Examination:* Order the steps in an intraoral examination.
- *15-2: Lesion Description—Reference File:* Identify six intraoral lesions using the decision tree matrix. This exercise also builds a decision tree matrix for the reference file.
- *15-3: Lesion Description—Audio:* Identify eight intraoral lesions by audio description.
- *15-4: Lesion Description—Maria Bjork:* Describe lesion and place information on patient chart for Maria Bjork.

- *15-5: Examination of the Lips and Labial Mucosa—Reference File:* Identify anatomical landmarks, and build a chart for the reference file.
- *15-6: Examination of the Lips and Labial Mucosa—Ann Cronin:* Identify normal oral structure on Ann Cronin.
- *15-7: Examination of the Lips and Labial Mucosa: Examination Technique—Reference File:* Identify anatomical landmarks, and build a chart for the reference file.
- *15-8: Examination of the Buccal Mucosa and Vestibular Folds—Reference File:* Identify anatomical landmarks, and build a chart for the reference file.
- *15-9 to 15-12: Examination of the Buccal Mucosa and Vestibular Folds:* Identify normal structures on William Johnston, Subra Mani, Elena Guri, and Adolfo Santana.
- *15-13 to 15-14: Examination of the Floor of the Mouth—Reference File:* Identify anatomical landmarks, and build a chart for the reference file.
- *15-15 to 15-16: Examination of the Tongue—Reference File:* Identify anatomical landmarks, and build a chart for the reference file.
- *15-17 to 15-18: Examination of the Tongue:* Identify normal structures on Elena Guri and Subra Mani.
- *15-19: Examination of the Hard and Soft Palates—Reference File:* Identify anatomical landmarks, and build a chart for the reference file.
- *15-20 to 15-21: Examination of the Hard and Soft Palates:* Identify normal structure on George Burkett and William Johnston.
- *15-22: Examination of the Oropharynx and Palatine Tonsils—Reference File:* Identify anatomical landmarks, and build a chart for the reference file.
- *15-23: Examination of the Oropharynx and Palatine Tonsils—George Burkett:* Identify normal structures on George Burkett.

Textbook

Review Case Study 15-1, Thorough Intraoral and Extraoral Examination, and the case applications. Consider the following questions regarding Case Study 15-1 at the beginning of the chapter. Using an intraoral findings charting form from your clinic, answer and document the following:

- What condition is presented as the lips are examined? Document on your form.
- What condition is presented as the buccal mucosa is examined? Document on your form.
- What condition is presented as the floor of the mouth is examined? Document on your form.
- What condition is presented as the tongue is examined? Document on you form.
- What condition is presented as the hard palate is examined? Document on your form.
- What condition is presented as the oropharynx is examined? Document on your form.

HOW do I perform these skills?

evolve

A printable version of this checklist is available on your Evolve Student Resources.

To provide a thorough intraoral examination, I will:

- ☐ Evaluate the patient's lips at rest.
- ☐ Examine the lips and vermillion border by slightly averting the lips manually to fully expose them to view.
- ☐ Examine the lips further with bidigital palpation, noting any abnormalities.
- ☐ Dry the mucosal surface of the buccal mucosa so that secretion of the accessory salivary glands of the cheek may be observed.
- ☐ Palpate the buccal mucosa.
- ☐ View the floor of the mouth.
- ☐ Palpate the floor of the mouth.
- ☐ Palpate the lingual aspect of the mandible.
- ☐ Examine and palpate the tongue.
- ☐ Examine the hard and soft palate.

- ☐ Palpate the hard and soft palate.
- ☐ Visually inspect the oropharynx and palatine tonsils.
- ☐ Palpate the tonsillar pillar and tonsillar bed (if possible).
- ☐ Document findings and procedure in chart.

HOW can I more effectively use this knowledge?

Critical Thinking Activities

Use the following worksheet to complete activitiy #5.

1. The tongue serves many oral functions. The one we think least about is the task of locating plaque. Place your tongue as far back on the buccal surface of your maxillary teeth as possible. What is the furthest tooth structure you can reach? Survey five classmates; check their response to this question. What problems in patient education could you foresee if tongue placement could not reach the distal of the most posterior tooth?
2. Survey five classmates for the following intraoral conditions, and tabulate your results:
   - Leukoedema
   - Linea alba
   - Palatine raphe
   - Salivary caruncles
   - Fordyce granules
   - Palatine tonsils
3. Describe the buccal mucosa of a patient with xerostomia. What do you think you would observe?
4. Working with a classmate, determine the best order in which to evaluate intraoral structures. Compare your order of examination with another group. Were any similarities present?
5. Using Worksheet #1, locate and describe the listed oral structures on three classmates. Note the subtle differences between these *normal* structures.

Worksheet #1

Use the following worksheet to complete Critical Thinking Activity #5.

	Patient 1	Patient 2	Patient 3
External Lip Region			
Nasolabial groove			
Philtrum			
Transitional zone			
Columella nasi			
Vermillion border			
Lateral commissures (angle)			
Labiomental groove			
Leukoedema (may or may not be present)			
Linea alba (may or may not be present)			
Parotid papilla			
Stensen's ducts			
Fordyce granules			
Palatoglossal arch or fold			
Palatopharyngeal arch or fold			
Uvula			
Posterior wall of pharynx			
Palatine tonsils			
Incisive papilla			
Palatine fovea			
Median palatine			
Raphae			
Palatal rugae			

Continued

	Patient 1	Patient 2	Patient 3
Dorsum			
Filiform papillae			
Fungiform papillae			
Median sulcus			
Circumvallate papillae			
Foramen cecum			
Sulcus terminalis			
Lingual tonsils			
Foliate papillae			
Plica fimbriata			
Ventral			
Lingual veins			
Lingual frenum			
Sublingual fold			
Plica lingualis			
Sublingual papilla or caruncle			
Vestibular Area			
Vestibular fold maxillary (mucolabial)			
Labial frenula			
Buccal or lateral frenula			
Alveolar mucosa (maxillary)			
Vestibular fold maxillary (mandibular)			

Chapter **15** **Intraoral Examination**

DO I have all the answers?

Review Questions

Check your answers against the Answer Key at the back of this Study Guide to assess what you have learned.

1. Mucosal tissue that appears wrinkled and filmy white but translucent when gently stretched taut is called which one of the following?
   a. Leukoplakia
   b. Candidiasis
   c. Leukoedema
   d. Erythema multiforme

2. Which one of the following describes a dense pad of tissue in the area just distal to the pterygomandibular fold behind the last mandibular molar?
   a. Retromolar pad
   b. Raphe
   c. Tuberosity
   d. Buccal mucosa

3. In an examination of the mucosal surface of the cheeks, drying the surface with gauze is best for which one of the following reasons?
   a. To increase patient comfort
   b. To gain a true picture of color
   c. To avoid slipping
   d. To observe secretion of accessory salivary glands

4. Fordyce granules can be found on which intraoral structure?
   a. On the hard palate
   b. In the buccal mucosa
   c. In the lip
   d. All of the above
   e. All but *a*

5. The sublingual caruncle holds the opening of which one of the following ducts?
   a. Palatine duct (Cusp of Carabelli Gland)
   b. Stenson's duct (Parotid Gland)
   c. Wharton's duct (Submandibular Gland)
   d. None of the above

6. The remnant of the thyroglossal duct, seen as a small pit at the apex of the sulcus terminalis, is termed which one of the following?
   a. Mental foramen
   b. Foramen cecum
   c. Sella turcica
   d. Median lingual sulcus

7. The armamentarium necessary to perform the intraoral examination includes which one of the following?
   a. Gauze
   b. Mouth mirror
   c. Air
   d. Overhead light
   e. All of the above

8. A white line running horizontally on the buccal mucosa is known as which one of the following terms?
   a. Leukoedema
   b. Candidiasis
   c. Lichen planus
   d. Linea alba
   e. None of the above

9. The small, spinelike projections covering most of the tongue's surface are which type of papilla?
   a. Filiform
   b. Fungiform
   c. Circumvallate
   d. Foliate

10. Palatine rugae are located on which portion of the palate?
    a. Anterior palate
    b. Palatine fovea
    c. Soft palate
    d. Vibrating line

WHERE do I go for more information or support?

evolve

For suggested web sites and agencies, additional readings and resources, and more chapter-specific information, please consult your Evolve Student Resources. Because of the ever-changing nature of the Internet, please keep in mind that web sites listed and their content may change.

CD-ROM

Reference files: Several of the exercises for Chapter 15 should be written to a reference file once you have completed them:

- *15-2: Lesion Description*
- *15-5: Examination of the Lips and Labial Mucosa*
- *15-7: Examination of the Lips and Labial Mucosa: Examination Technique*
- *15-8: Examination of the Buccal Mucosa and Vestibular Folds: Examination Technique*
- *15-14 to 15-15: Examination of the Floor of the Mouth*
- *15-15 to 15-18: Examination of the Tongue*
- *15-19: Examination of the Hard and Soft Palates*
- *15-22: Examination of the Oropharynx and Palatine Tonsils*

Charts created for these exercises can be printed out to keep with your class materials.

HOW can I keep track of my progress toward competence?

As an ongoing picture of progress, record and monitor clinical experiences relating to Chapter 15 content in your Portfolio.

Self-Reflection

On a regular basis, review these experiences (with a faculty member). Identify strengths, weaknesses (not just numbers), and changes that you would incorporate into your clinical care plan now that you have had these experiences.

16 Periodontal Examination

WHY do I need to know about the Periodontal Examination?

The dental hygienist is uniquely educated to perform a comprehensive periodontal examination and is frequently referred to as the periodontal co-therapist on the oral healthcare team.

WHAT will I be able to do with this knowledge?

1. Describe the roles of plaque biofilm and other local etiologic factors in periodontal diseases.
2. Identify the components of a periodontal assessment, their appearance in health and disease, and their significance.
3. Chart an involved periodontal condition, using the correct charting notations.
4. Interpret the periodontal findings from a chart (i.e., correctly read a periodontal chart), and discuss the ramifications.
5. Explain the interrelationships and suggested interrelationships between periodontitis and systemic diseases as presently reported in the scientific literature.
6. Identify those patients who have periodontitis or those who are at risk for periodontitis.

HOW do I prepare myself to transfer this knowledge to patient care?

 Go to Chapter 16 content on your CD-ROM or search for the following terms:
   Periodontal Examination
   Gingiva
   Furcation
   Mobility
   Attachment Loss
   Periodontal
   Plaque Biofilm

CD Exercises

- *16-1: Anatomical Landmarks of the Periodontium— Reference File:* Locate and label 11 periodontal landmarks. This exercise also builds a chart for your reference file.
- *16-2: Visual Characteristics of the Gingiva:* Describe six gingival conditions.

- *16-3: Descriptive Characteristics of the Gingiva:* Describe gingival conditions (select correct oral image from audio description).
- *16-4 to 16-5: Visual Characteristics of the Gingiva:* Describe gingival conditions from patient files for Adolfo Santana and William Johnston.
- *16-6: Calculation of Attachment Loss:* Calculate attachment loss in a given scenario.
- *16-7: Components of the Periodontal Examination:* Through an audio reading, build an entire periodontal charting (four separate quadrants).
- *16-8: Components of the Periodontal Examination— Ann Cronin:* Complete a quadrant of charting on Ann Cronin.
- *16-9: Exploration of Furcations— Reference File:* Match the correct classification symbol to classification. This exercise also builds a chart for your reference file.
- *16-10: Exploration of Furcations:* Match photographs of furcation involvement to classification.
- *16-11 to 16-12: Exploration of Furcations:* Identify furcation involvement on George Burkett and Elena Guri.
- *16-13: Detection of Mobility—Reference File:* Match the correct symbol to the classification. This exercise also builds a chart for your reference file.
- *16-14: Detection of Mobility:* Identify classification of mobility from animation.
- *16-15. Assessment of Plaque and Calculus—Terrence Zellar:* Assess microbial plaque from patient records for Terrence Zellar.

Textbook

Review Case Study 16-1, Completing the Periodontal Examination, and consider your answers to the case applications.

For important concepts and application of knowledge, review tables, figures, and boxed sections of the book.

The following chapter elements may be especially helpful for clinical transfer and may be used as a clinical reference:

- Figures 16-3 through 16-6, 16-10 through 16-12, 16-16, 16-19, 16-23, 16-26, and 16-27
- Boxes 16-1 through 16-4 and 16-6
- Tables 16-1, 16-2, and 16-8

83

HOW do I perform these skills?

evolve

A printable version of this checklist is available on your Evolve Student Resources.

To provide a thorough periodontal examination, I will:

☐ Describe the visual characteristics of the gingiva.

☐ Measure the location of the free gingival margin or recession in relation to the cementoenamel junction.

☐ Measure and record probe depths.

☐ Calculate attachment loss.

☐ Measure keratinized or attached gingiva.

☐ Detect and record bleeding on probing.

☐ Detect and record suppuration.

☐ Explore furcations.

☐ Detect and record mobility.

☐ Assess plaque biofilm and calculus accumulations.

☐ Document findings and procedure in chart.

HOW can I more effectively use this knowledge?

Critical Thinking Activities

1. Review clinical photographs, and describe the characteristics of the gingiva.
2. Practice calculating attachment loss using probe depths and recession readings.
3. Complete a comprehensive periodontal charting on a peer or patient.
4. Record periodontal findings for a student clinician.
5. Review patient cases, and identify the American Academy of Periodontology's periodontal classification. Provide rationales for your responses.
6. Given sites of bleeding, plaque biofilm, and gingival inflammation, calculate an index for each.

DO I have all the answers?

Review Questions

Check your answers against the Answer Key at the back of this Study Guide to assess what you have learned. Questions 1 through 7 refer to Case Study 16-1.

1. Which one of the following is the most appropriate periodontal diagnosis for Mrs. Bozenski?
   a. Aggressive periodontitis and early-onset periodontitis
   b. Chronic periodontitis and adult periodontitis
   c. Periodontitis associated with systemic disease
   d. Refractory periodontitis
   e. Not enough information present to make a diagnosis

2. A secondary diagnosis may include which one of the following?
   a. Pregnancy-associated gingivitis
   b. Postmenopausal periodontitis
   c. Occlusal trauma
   d. Aspirin-associated bleeding on probing
   e. Inderal-induced gingival overgrowth

3. During an examination of the pocket on the mesiolabial of the maxillary right canine, with 25 gm of probing force, the tip of the probe will *most likely* do which one of the following?
   a. Stop at the base of the histologic pocket.
   b. Penetrate into but not through the junctional epithelium.
   c. Penetrate through the junctional epithelium into the underlying connective tissue.
   d. Penetrate through the epithelium and connective tissue and stop when the tip touches the crest of the alveolar bone.
   e. None of the above will occur.

4. Which one of the following is the instrument of choice with which to examine furcations?
   a. Moffitt-Maryland periodontal probe
   b. No. 23 Shepherd's hook explorer
   c. Pigtail explorer
   d. 2N Nabers probe

5. Which one of the following is the furcation involvement on the mesial of the maxillary left first molar?
   a. Class I
   b. Class II
   c. Class III
   d. Class IV

6. Which one of the following describes the meaning of the mobility measurement of the maxillary left first molar?
   a. The tooth has three roots.
   b. The tooth is depressible and has lateral mobility.
   c. The tooth is stable in all three dimensions (x, y, and z).
   d. There is nothing to worry about because mobility is measured on a scale of 1 to 10.

7. Based on the medical history presented for Mrs. Bozenski, antibiotic prophylaxis must have been administered before she underwent any type of dental treatment.
   a. True
   b. False

8. Which one of the following teeth has the greatest *radiographic* furcation involvement?
   a. Mandibular right first molar
   b. Mandibular left first molar
   c. Maxillary right first molar
   d. Maxillary left first molar

WHERE do I go for more information or support?

For suggested web sites and agencies, additional readings and resources, and more chapter-specific information, please consult your Evolve Student Resources. Because of the ever-changing nature of the Internet, please keep in mind that web sites listed and their content may change.

CD-ROM

Reference files: Several of the exercises for Chapter 16 should be written to a reference file once you have completed them:

- *16-1: Anatomical Landmarks of the Periodontium*
- *16-3: Descriptive Characteristics of the Gingiva*
- *16-9: Exploration of Furcations*
- *16-13: Detection of Mobility*

HOW can I keep track of my progress toward competence?

As an ongoing picture of progress, record and monitor clinical experiences relating to Chapter 16 content in your Portfolio.

Self-Reflection

On a regular basis, review these experiences (with a faculty member). Identify strengths, weaknesses (not just numbers), and changes that you would incorporate into your clinical care plan now that you have had these experiences.

17 Hard Tissue Examination

WHY do I need to know about Hard Tissue Examination?

An accurate dental charting provides a picture of the patient's mouth with existing restorations, pathologic conditions, and other clinical information such as missing, rotated, and impacted teeth. This record is significant for future dental needs and for forensics for patient identification. The dental hygienist is often in a position to examine and record clinical findings and to update chartings periodically. Recognition of clinical conditions and knowledge of charting these conditions is essential for thorough patient documentation and treatment.

WHAT will I be able to do with this knowledge?

1. Use a number of different comprehensive charting systems to assess the oral health of new patients and supportive care patients.
2. Be familiar with the different tooth-numbering systems.
3. Use proper infection control during performance of charting procedures.
4. Use the traditional GV Black Caries Classification System to chart existing conditions.
5. Be familiar with new classification systems for carious lesions.
6. Use different charting symbols that represent existing conditions, such as early carious lesions before cavitation, dental caries requiring restoration, missing teeth, partially erupted teeth, malposed teeth, existing dental restorations, erosion, abrasion, attrition, abfraction, enamel cracking, and cusp fracture.
7. Define *dental caries* and related terms.
8. Recognize the signs of dental caries, including carious lesions, in varying stages of development.
9. Recognize the signs of arrested versus active carious lesions.
10. Recognize the signs of recurrent or secondary dental caries.
11. Recognize different stages of carious lesions and different dental restorations on a radiograph.
12. Classify occlusion with Angle's Classification System, measuring overbite and overjet and identifying the signs of occlusal trauma.

HOW do I prepare myself to transfer this knowledge to patient care?

 Go to Chapter 17 content on your CD-ROM or search for "Hard Tissue."

CD Exercises

- *17-1: Comprehensive Hard Tissue Charting:* From an audio reading, chart oral conditions for Maria Bjork.
- *17-2: Comprehensive Hard Tissue Charting—Eva Bjork:* Complete a quadrant of charting from photographs and radiographs for Eva Bjork.
- *17-3: Comprehensive Hard Tissue Charting—Adolfo Santana:* Note oral conditions for Adolfo Santana based on charts and records.
- *17-4: Other Conditions that Modify Teeth:* Identify photographs of erosion, abrasion, attrition, and abfraction.
- *17-5: Occlusal Analysis—Terrence Zellar:* Classify occlusion for Terrence Zellar using intraoral photographs.
- *17-6: Angle's Classification—Ann Cronin, George Burkett, William Johnston, Maria Bjork, Subra Mani:* Identify Angle's classification system—patient cases.

Textbook

Review Case Study 17-1, Examination and Recording of Dental Findings, and the case applications

HOW do I perform these skills?

evolve

A printable version of this checklist is available on your Evolve Student Resources.
To provide a thorough hard tissue examination, I will:
  ☐ Chart existing hard tissue conditions.
  ☐ Chart dental caries.
  ☐ Document Angle's classification of occlusion.
  ☐ Document findings and procedure in chart.

HOW can I more effectively use this knowledge?

Critical Thinking Activities

On a patient charting form, record the following conditions:
- A 2-mm diastema between teeth #9 and #10
- A four-unit bridge between teeth #11 and #14 (abutment teeth: #11 and #14; pontics: #12 and #13)

- Tooth #14: All gold extending to the cementoenamel junction (CEJ)
- Tooth #13: Porcelain on the facial extending from the CEJ to the central groove on the occlusal; gold from the central groove to the lingual margin, which is at the CEJ
- Tooth #12: Porcelain on the facial extending from the CEJ to the central groove on the occlusal; gold from the central groove to the lingual margin, which is at the CEJ
- Tooth #11: Porcelain on the facial and lingual extending from the CEJ to halfway down the lingual surface; gold on the other half of the lingual surface
- Tooth #2: Acrylic temporary crown covering the entire crown to 1 mm below the CEJ
- Tooth #19: Occlusal amalgam with an ideal outline form with dental caries that can be seen clinically along at the margins of the distal pit
- Tooth #5: Dental caries (not to the dentinoenamel junction [DEJ]) that can be seen radiographically and clinically under the distal contact
- Tooth #7: Completed single-root endodontics (seen radiographically) with a lingual pit amalgam
- Tooth #30: Occlusal composite 2 mm wide along central groove between mesial and distal pits
- Tooth #32: Horizontally impacted and completely covered by tissue
- Tooth #8: Distal incisal fracture with piece of tooth missing

DO I have all the answers?

Review Questions

Check your answers against the Answer Key at the back of this Study Guide to assess what you have learned.

1. All of the following statements are true *except* which one?
   a. Sensitivity is the ability to correctly identify health or the absence of carious lesions.
   b. A #1.2 lesion is Mount and Hume's classification of a medium-sized cavity in the top of the tooth.
   c. E0 classification means that no lesions are visible.
   d. Secondary dental caries is more likely to occur at gingival margins than occlusal margins (especially in amalgams).
   e. Bacteria-filled dentin is called *infected dentin.*

2. All *except* which one of the following are limitations involving the use of an explorer to detect occlusal caries?
   a. Use of an explorer to detect occlusal caries is only 60% accurate.
   b. It can transfer bacteria to other sites.
   c. It can damage intact surfaces.
   d. It can give false-positive results.
   e. It can give false-negative results.

3. Which one of the following statements best describes the process of attrition?
   a. The wearing of the tooth substance by exogenous material forced over the surface by incisive, masticatory, or tooth-cleaning functions
   b. The superficial loss of dental hard tissue because of a chemical process not involving bacteria
   c. Tooth wear caused by tooth-to-tooth contact without the presence of exogenous material
   d. Flexure at the cervical region of the tooth, causing loss of mineral
   e. None of the above

4. Which one of the following statements best characterizes abrasion?
   a. The wearing of the tooth substance by exogenous material forced over the surface by incisive, masticatory, or tooth-cleaning functions
   b. The superficial loss of dental hard tissue because of a chemical process not involving bacteria
   c. Tooth wear caused by tooth-to-tooth contact without the presence of exogenous material
   d. Flexure at the cervical region of the tooth, causing loss of mineral
   e. None of the above

5. White spot lesions are the result of which one of the following occurrences?
   a. Too much fluoride in water
   b. Too much abrasive in dentifrice
   c. More topical fluoride treatments than warranted
   d. Change in refractive index because of demineralization
   e. Infusion of exogenous proteins into enamel surface

WHERE do I go for more information or support?

evolve

For suggested web sites and agencies, additional readings and resources, and more chapter-specific information, please consult your Evolve Student Resources. Because of the ever-changing nature of the Internet, please keep in mind that web sites listed and their content may change.

CD-ROM

Reference files: As you work through the CD-ROM exercises, you should be able to print reference files and add them to your class materials. No specific reference files apply to this chapter.

HOW can I keep track of my progress toward competence?

As an ongoing picture of progress, record and monitor clinical experiences relating to Chapter 17 content in your Portfolio.

Self-Reflection

On a regular basis, review these experiences (with a faculty member). Identify strengths, weaknesses (not just numbers), and changes that you would incorporate into your clinical care plan now that you have had these experiences.

18 Radiographic Evaluation and Intraoral Photographic Imaging

WHY do I need to know about Radiographic Evaluation and Intraoral Photographic Imaging?

The dental hygienist should evaluate the patient before the dentist determines the appropriate radiographs to be ordered. Points to consider in this evaluation include the patient's medical and dental history, current chief complaint, previous radiographs, or other clinical information.

WHAT will I be able to do with this knowledge?

1. Establish the appropriate radiographic series for a given patient based on the guidelines for prescribing dental radiographs, including the ALARA (as low as reasonably achievable) principle.
2. List the various types of intraoral and extraoral radiographic projections and their uses.
3. Identify the factors that contribute to the poor diagnostic quality of radiographs.
4. Discuss the fundamentals of digital imaging and cone-beam technology.
5. Recognize and understand the use of intraoral photographic imaging (IPI) in dentistry
6. Become familiar with the types of IPI equipment and accessories required for the documentation of intraoral anatomy.
7. Use radiographic imaging and IPI to gather assessment information and develop an appropriate care plan.

HOW do I prepare myself to transfer this knowledge to patient care?

 Go to Chapter 18 content on your CD-ROM or search for "Radiographs" or "Intraoral Imaging."

CD Exercises

- *18-1: Types of Intraoral and Extraoral Images—Ann Cronin:* Evaluate radiographs from Ann Cronin's file.
- *18-2 to 18-5: Intraoral Photographic Imaging:* Evaluate the use of intraoral imaging on Eva Bjork, Maria Bjork, Terrence Zellar, and Subra Mani.

Textbook

Review the case studies in the text book.

- Which radiographic series would you recommend for Mr. J., and what is your rationale for this decision?
- Which radiographic series would you recommend for Mrs. K., and what is your rationale for this decision?

- In Case Study 18-3, can you identify any technique errors other than the ones described?

HOW do I perform these skills?

evolve

A printable version of this checklist is available on your Evolve Student Resources.
To provide a thorough radiographic evaluation, I will:
- ☐ Select the appropriate radiographic series based on patient need.
- ☐ Assess radiographic quality.
- ☐ Retake radiographs as appropriate.
- ☐ Describe conditions present on each film.
- ☐ Develop a treatment plan with the dentist.
- ☐ Document x-ray film exposure, including retakes, in the chart.

HOW can I more effectively use this knowledge?

Critical Thinking Activities

1. Given a case history and clinical findings, determine the type and number of radiographs to be exposed according to the guidelines presented in Table 18-1.
2. Discuss with classmates the ways your school's radiology clinic follows the ALARA principle.
3. What is the recommended practice for handling a patient who refuses to have dental radiographs exposed? Role-play with classmates, alternating between the radiographer and the patient.
4. Compare two radiographic series: one series produced with dental film and one series produced through digital imaging. Look for differences in film contrast and density, as well as the ability to view dental caries, periodontal disease, or both.
5. Explain the advantages and disadvantages between digital imaging and conventional film to a patient.
6. Discuss clinical situations in which cone-beam imaging would be a valuable adjunct to existing radiographs.
7. Take a series of photographs using film in a 35 mm camera followed by a series of photographs using a digital camera. Compare the colors of the oral tissues and the amount of glare or other artifacts.

8. Work in groups of three with a 35 mm camera and a digital camera (one student acts as the patient, one operates the camera, and one places the intraoral mirrors and retractors). Discuss each task and compare the roles.

9. Practice the placement of the intraoral video camera wand to achieve images of all areas of the mouth.

DO I have all the answers?

Review Questions

Check your answers against the Answer Key at the back of this Study Guide to assess what you have learned.

1. Identify the primary reason for exposure of bite-wing images.
   a. Identification of periodontal disease
   b. Detection of dental caries
   c. Viewing of periapical regions
   d. Evaluation of growth and development

2. Incorrect horizontal angulation on a bite-wing image appears as which of the following?
   a. Overlapping of anatomy
   b. Elongation of structures
   c. Foreshortening of structures
   d. A darkened image

3. When comparing digital imaging with conventional radiography, the pixel may be compared with which of the following?
   a. Processing solutions
   b. Silver halide crystals
   c. Emulsion
   d. Film

4. Identify a disadvantage of digital radiography.
   a. Initial set-up cost
   b. Infection control issues
   c. Size and dimension of the intraoral sensor
   d. All of the above

5. Three-dimensional images are available for the dental professional through which of the following?
   a. Cone-beam imaging
   b. Panoramic radiography
   c. Extraoral images
   d. All of the above

6. In Figure 18-1, identify the restorative material seen in the patient's maxillary right quadrant.
   a. Gold bridge
   b. Amalgam restorations
   c. Porcelain-fused-to-metal bridge
   d. Partial removable denture

7. In Figure 18-1, identify the radiopacity seen inferior to the mandibular incisors.
   a. Genial tubercles
   b. Lingual foramen
   c. Mandibular tori
   d. Mylohyoid ridge

8. In Figure 18-1, identify the error seen in the maxillary central incisor projection.
   a. Cone cut
   b. Incorrect packet placement
   c. Reversed film
   d. Incorrect vertical angulation

9. In Figure 18-1, the inverted Y seen superior to the maxillary canines represents the intersection of which two structures?
   a. Maxillary sinus and nasal cavity
   b. Zygomatic process and maxillary sinus
   c. Nasal cavity and lateral fossa
   d. Nasal septum and median palatal suture

10. When selecting an intraoral photographic imaging (IPI) system appropriate for use in a dental office, the clinician should consider which of the following?
    a. Cost of the system
    b. Clarity of the images produced
    c. Technical support and ease of use
    d. All of the above

11. The recommended focal length for clinical photography is 105 mm. This length provides a better working distance for the clinician and comfort for the patient.
    a. Both statements are true.
    b. Both statements are false.
    c. The first statement is true; the second statement is false.
    d. The first statement is false; the second statement is true.

WHERE do I go for more information or support?

evolve

For suggested web sites and agencies, additional readings and resources, and more chapter-specific information, please consult your Evolve Student Resources. Because of the ever-changing nature of the Internet, please keep in mind that web sites listed and their content may change.

CD-ROM

Reference files: As you work through the CD-ROM exercises, you should be able to print reference files and add them to your class materials. No specific reference files apply to this chapter.

HOW can I keep track of my progress toward competence?

As an ongoing picture of progress, record and monitor clinical experiences relating to Chapter 18 content in your Portfolio.

Self-Reflection

On a regular basis, review these experiences (with a faculty member). Identify strengths, weaknesses (not just numbers), and changes that you would incorporate into your clinical care plan now that you have had these experiences.

19 Nutritional Assessment

WHY do I need to know about Nutritional Assessment?

Nutrition has a tremendous affect on both oral and overall general health. Dental hygienists must recognize the relationship among dental health, disease prevention and wellness, and nutrition.

WHAT will I be able to do with this knowledge?

1. Discuss dental conditions associated with nutrient imbalances.
2. Outline conditions in the oral cavity that inhibit food intake.
3. Describe conditions under which fermentable carbohydrates are cariogenic or noncariogenic.
4. Assess the dental patient to determine whether nutritional care is needed and the type and amount of nutritional intervention that is required.
5. Develop strategies to provide the highest-quality health care that will correct the diet-related dental situation.
6. Evaluate the effectiveness of nutritional intervention in a dental patient.

HOW do I prepare myself to transfer this knowledge to patient care?

 Go to Chapter 19 content on your CD-ROM or search for "Intraoral Exam" or "Oral Anatomy."

CD Exercises
- *19-1 to 19-2: Effects of Nutrition on the Oral Cavity:* Complete an assessment of a 24-hour diet recall for Maria Bjork and Elena Guri.
- Note: All patients on the CD-ROM have fully developed 24-hour nutritional assessments for additional student assignment.

Textbook
Review Case Study 19-1, Effects of Nutrition on Oral Health, and the case applications. Consider the following questions after reading the applications:
- What recommendations might you make for John to remove soda and mints from his diet?
- John has a 1-day diet summary. Would you recommend a 3- or 7-day food record? What difference might you see?

HOW do I perform these skills?

evolve

A printable version of this checklist is available on your Evolve Student Resources.
To provide a thorough nutritional assessment and utilization, I will:
- ☐ Identify any dental anomalies associated with nutrient imbalances.
- ☐ Identify any oral complications preventing proper nutrition.
- ☐ Educate patient on diet and dietary habits contributing to dental caries.
- ☐ Review the health history for risk factors suggestive of nutritional problems.
- ☐ Perform extraoral and intraoral examinations.
- ☐ Review findings from standard saliva tests, plaque biofilm–control indices, and dental caries risk-assessment activities.
- ☐ Record a patient's food intake.
- ☐ Analyze dietary intake data.
- ☐ Develop a personalized intervention strategy.
- ☐ Determine a reevaluation schedule.
- ☐ Document process in chart.

HOW can I more effectively use this knowledge?

Critical Thinking Activities
Use the following worksheet to complete activity #1.
1. Using Worksheet #1, write down everything you consume for 3 consecutive days, including 1 weekend day. Determine your calorie level using "My Pyramid Plan" at www.mypyramid.gov, and obtain the MyPyramid Worksheet for your specific calorie range. Compare your intake with the MyPyramid Food Guidance System. In which groups are you within range? Which groups do you need to modify? List at least two realistic changes that you can make to improve your dietary intake.
2. Compare your lifestyle and eating with the USDA's 2005 Dietary Guidelines for Americans. Which guidelines do you follow? Which guidelines can you improve?
3. Interview a partner to establish his or her intake from the previous day, and enter the information in a food diary

(see the Evolve site for a food diary worksheet). Which questions did you need to ask to clarify the person's food intake? Circle the fermentable carbohydrates in red, and determine which aspects of each meal or snack are cariogenic.

4. Poll the class members at a local high school to establish the average number of sodas, sports drinks, bottled or canned teas, specialty coffee drinks, and milk they consume each day. Provide education to the class concerning the nutritional and dental issues related to beverage intake. Brainstorm appropriate substitutions or alternative behaviors. To reinforce the topic, place an extracted tooth in soda for a week before the presentation and share the results with the class.

Worksheet #1

Use the following form to complete Critical Thinking Activity #1.

DAY 1

Food Group	Recommended Servings	Actual	Comparison
Bread, cereal, rice, pasta	6-11	_____	_____
Fruit	2-4	_____	_____
Vegetable	3-5	_____	_____
Milk, yogurt, cheese	4	_____	_____
Meat, poultry, fish, dry beans, eggs, nuts	2-3	_____	_____
Fats, oils	Sparingly	_____	_____
Sweets	Sparingly	_____	_____

DAY 2

Food Group	Recommended Servings	Actual	Comparison
Bread, cereal, rice, pasta	6-11	_____	_____
Fruit	2-4	_____	_____
Vegetable	3-5	_____	_____
Milk, yogurt, cheese	4	_____	_____
Meat, poultry, fish, dry beans, eggs, nuts	2-3	_____	_____
Fats, oils	Sparingly	_____	_____
Sweets	Sparingly	_____	_____

DAY 3

Food Group	Recommended Servings	Actual	Comparison
Bread, cereal, rice, pasta	6-11	_____	_____
Fruit	2-4	_____	_____
Vegetable	3-5	_____	_____
Milk, yogurt, cheese	4	_____	_____
Meat, poultry, fish, dry beans, eggs, nuts	2-3	_____	_____
Fats, oils	Sparingly	_____	_____
Sweets	Sparingly	_____	_____

Chapter **19** **Nutritional Assessment**

DO I have all the answers?

Review Questions

Check your answers against the Answer Key at the back of this Study Guide to assess what you have learned.

1. Which one of the following choices provides the most reliable data collection regarding nutritional intake?
   a. 24-hour recall
   b. 3- to 7-day diet survey
   c. Evaluation of food textures over 1 week
   d. Evaluation of times of carbohydrate consumption

2. Which one of the following groups of foods is considered protective to the oral cavity against the development of dental caries?
   a. Carrots, broccoli, foods with saccharin
   b. Nuts, cream cheese, foods with xylitol
   c. Milk, fruit juice, raisins
   d. Fish, poultry, legumes, peanut butter

3. Positive responses to which one of the following items on a health history might indicate xerostomia?
   a. Depression
   b. Liquid diet
   c. Diabetes
   d. Medications
   e. All of the above

4. Which one of the following groups of individuals is at nutritional risk?
   a. Infants
   b. Older adults with osteoporosis
   c. Alcoholics
   d. Pregnant women
   e. All of the above

5. Posteruptively, which one of the following choices is the most significant dietary influence on the development of dental caries?
   a. Fermentable carbohydrate content of the diet
   b. Overall vitamin content of the diet
   c. Mineral content of the diet
   d. Protein content of the diet

6. In which one of the following ways can inadequate nutritional intake contribute to periodontal disease?
   a. Delays in wound healing
   b. Interference with collagen maintenance and repair
   c. Increases in bleeding on probing
   d. All of the above
   e. Only *a* and *b*

7. Once consumed, a fermentable carbohydrate eaten alone can produce a drop in salivary pH in approximately which one of the following amounts of time?
   a. 2 to 4 minutes
   b. 10 minutes
   c. 20 to 30 minutes
   d. 1 hour
   e. 1 day

8. Once plaque pH has been affected by the resulting acid production of oral bacteria, how long will the lowered (acidic) pH remain before being buffered by the saliva?
   a. 2 to 4 minutes
   b. 10 minutes
   c. 20 to 30 minutes
   d. 1 hour
   e. 1 day

9. Which one of the following statements concerning nutrition is *true*?
   a. Each dental hygienist should develop a list of cariogenic foods as a handout for patients to avoid.
   b. Nonnutritive sweeteners produce dental caries.
   c. Nutrient intake has a significant affect on salivary composition.
   d. Sugar alcohols are never cariogenic.
   e. All of the above.
   f. None of the above.

10. Which one of the following numbers identifies a plaque biofilm pH capable of promoting demineralization?
    a. 5.5
    b. 7.0
    c. 7.5
    d. 10.0
    e. 12.5

WHERE do I go for more information or support?

 evolve

For suggested web sites and agencies, additional readings and resources, and more chapter-specific information, please consult your Evolve Student Resources. Because of the ever-changing nature of the Internet, please keep in mind that web sites listed and their content may change.

CD CD-ROM

Reference files: As you work through the CD-ROM exercises, you should be able to print reference files and add them to your class materials. No specific reference files apply to this chapter.

HOW can I keep track of my progress toward competence?

As an ongoing picture of progress, record and monitor clinical experiences relating to Chapter 19 content in your Portfolio.

Self-Reflection

On a regular basis, review these experiences (with a faculty member). Identify strengths, weaknesses (not just numbers), and changes that you would incorporate into your clinical care plan now that you have had these experiences.

20 Oral Risk Assessment and Intervention Planning

WHY do I need to know about Oral Risk Assessment and Intervention Planning?

Dental hygienists often provide treatment, service, and care for individuals in a way these patients may have never before experienced. In Case Study 20-1, consider both the complexity and the opportunity to change a lifetime of dental neglect.

WHAT will I be able to do with this knowledge?

1. Determine a working definition for the following terms: intervention, oral risk assessment, prevention, risk, and risk assessment.
2. Compare and contrast a patient-specific approach to care with a standardized routine.
3. Give examples of patient-centered oral care.
4. Cite examples of therapeutic intervention in dentistry.
5. Cite examples of prevention strategies in dentistry.
6. Cite examples of when therapeutic intervention and prevention overlap in dentistry.
7. Describe the benefits of oral risk assessment to individualizing preventive and therapeutic strategies.
8. Develop a clinical goal, therapeutic intervention, and evaluation measure based on a given oral risk concern.

HOW do I prepare myself to transfer this knowledge to patient care?

 Go to Chapter 20 content on your CD-ROM or search for "Oral Risk Assessment."

CD Exercises

- *20-1 to 20-9: Case Summary:* Following a narrated and animated demonstration of the oral risk assessment process, complete any or all patient assessments as desired or assigned.

Textbook

Review Case Study 20-1, Therapeutic Intervention with Risk Assessment, presented at the beginning of the chapter. In the third paragraph, questions are posed. Respond to the questions presented.

HOW do I perform these skills?

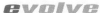 *evolve*

A printable version of this checklist is available on your Evolve Student Resources.

To implement the oral risk assessment system successfully, I will:
- ☐ Review assessment data.
- ☐ Analyze all data for oral risk concerns.
- ☐ Plan the goals of intervention therapy.
- ☐ Plan the goals of personalized prevention strategies.
- ☐ Evaluate or reevaluate outcomes of clinical dental hygiene therapy and recommended alternatives as appropriate.

HOW can I more effectively use this knowledge?

Critical Thinking Activities

Use the following worksheet to complete your activities.

1. Together with a classmate, fill out the prevention survey in Worksheet #1. In a role-playing format, perform Step 1 of the oral risk assessment system, using the oral risk assessment worksheet. Did you overlook any pertinent findings from this step? Did any biological, psychologic, or sociologic elements come to light that might influence the therapeutic and intervention strategies?
2. Make a list of all therapeutic intervention strategies that you perform as a dental hygienist. Determine whether each strategy acts strictly as an intervention, a prevention, or both.
3. Using Worksheet #1, perform Step 2 of an oral risk assessment with a student partner. What types of oral concerns can you clinically document? Which types are potential oral concerns?
4. Go on line and review the Surgeon General's Report *Oral Health in America* (see the suggested agencies and web sites listed on the Evolve site). In what ways does the oral risk assessment system support a more holistic approach to oral care?
5. If you are a first-year student, select a second-year student with whom to work. Ask to review the dental records of a patient that your partner is currently treating. After completing Steps 1 and 2 of the oral risk assessment system using only the dental records provided, complete Step 3 using Worksheet #1. Determine the clinical goal, therapeutic intervention, and evaluation method for each oral risk concern noted. Would this process have been more thorough with a prevention survey?

Worksheet #1—Oral Risk Assessment Worksheet

Patient Name_____   Date_____

I

REVIEW

Health History	Medications & Dose Duration
❑ Cardiovascular (heart)	(prescription and OTC)
❑ Central nervous system (nerves)	
❑ Endocrine (endocrine glands)	
❑ Gastrointestinal (stomach, intestines)	
❑ Genitourinary (sex organs, urinary tract)	
❑ Head, eyes, ears, nose, throat	
❑ Hematologic (blood)	
❑ Integumentary (skin)	
❑ Musculoskeletal (muscles, bones, joints)	
❑ Psychologic	
❑ Respiratory	

Vital Signs BP   /   Pulse

PREVENTION SURVEY

Dental History

❑ Sensitive teeth	❑ Sore jaw	❑ Toothache	❑ Sore gums	❑ Clenching
❑ Bleeding gums	❑ Difficulty chewing	❑ Filling fell out	❑ Dry mouth	❑ Grinding
❑ Bad breath	❑ Burning sensation		❑ Abscess	❑ Swollen face
❑ Swelling inside mouth	❑ Tartar buildup	❑ Yellowing teeth	❑ Difficulty swallowing	
❑ Adequate OH time	❑ Anxiety/Pain	❑ Oral self-care difficulty		

Oral Health Products:

Fluoride History

❑ Fluoridated water	❑ Away from home >4 days/week	❑ Oral rinse w/fluoride
❑ Water filter	❑ Bottled juice	Child:
❑ Bottled water	❑ Fluoridated dentifrice	❑ In daycare w/out fluoride ❑ Supplements

Behaviors

❑ Annual physical	❑ Balance work/relaxation	❑ Tobacco use	❑ Exercise
❑ Follows medical advice	❑ Eating habits controlled	❑ Alcohol use	
❑ Follows dental advice	❑ Increased stress	❑ Caffeine use	

Diet Survey   ❑ Carbohydrate/Sucrose intake (excessive/moderate/minimal)

Beliefs

❑ Understands oral status	❑ Values prevention
❑ Wants product recommendations	❑ Open to change ❑ Feels in control of oral condition

Clinical and Radiographic Findings

Intraoral/Extraoral Examination	❑ Within normal limits		❑ See chart
Caries	❑ Coronal	❑ Interproximal	❑ Root surface

Restorations/Prosthetics

Restorations	❑ Amalgam	❑ Composite	❑ Crowns/inlays/onlays	❑ Bridges
Dentures	❑ Complete	❑ Partial		

Periodontium

❑ Recession	❑ Plaque ❑ Bleeding on probing	❑ Loss of attached gingiva	❑ Pockets <3mm
❑ Mucogingival defects			

Occlusion/TMJ	❑ Traumatic occlusion	❑ Crepitus	
Bone Loss	❑ <25%	❑ 25-50%	❑ Horizontal	❑ Vertical

Continued

Chapter **20 Oral Risk Assessment and Intervention Planning**

II

ANALYZE
Oral Risk Concerns

At risk for   **Clinically Evident**

Hard Tissues

At risk for		Clinically Evident
❑	Abrasion/Attrition/Erosion	❑
❑	Bone Loss	❑
❑	Bruxism/Occlusal Trauma	❑
❑	Calculus	❑
❑	Caries: coronal/interproximal	❑
❑	Caries: root surface	❑
❑	Chipped broken teeth	❑
❑	Extrinsic staining	❑
❑	Fluorosis	❑
❑	Intrinsic staining	❑
❑	Malaligned teeth	❑
❑	Mobile teeth	❑
❑	Sensitive teeth	❑
❑	Trauma	❑
❑	Other	❑

Soft Tissues

At risk for		Clinically Evident
❑	Abscess: carious	❑
❑	Abscess: periodontal	❑
❑	Atrophic ulcer	❑
❑	Aphthous ulcer	❑
❑	Burning tongue/mouth	❑
❑	Candidiasis	❑
❑	Ecchymosis	❑
❑	Gingival recession	❑
❑	Gingival hyperplasia	❑
❑	Gingivitis	❑
❑	Herpetic lesions	❑
❑	Increased plaque	❑
❑	Leukoplakia	❑
❑	Lichen planus	❑
❑	Oral cancer	❑
❑	Periodontal disease	❑
❑	Petechiae	❑
❑	Salivation – increased	❑
❑	Salivation – decreased	❑
❑	Trauma	❑
❑	Xerostomia	❑
❑	Other_____	❑

Consult   **Referral**

Consult		Referral
❑	Consultation with physician	❑
❑	Consultation with dental specialist	❑

III

PLAN		
Clinical Goals	**Therapeutic Intervention**	**Patient Goals**

Chapter **20** **Oral Risk Assessment and Intervention Planning**

Review Questions

Check your answers against the Answer Key at the back of this Study Guide to assess what you have learned.
Questions 5 through 7 and question 9 refer to Case Study 20-1.

1. A patient-specific approach to oral care includes which one of the following approaches?
   a. Following a standard therapeutic intervention, individualizing the prevention aspects based principally on current patient knowledge
   b. Gaining an understanding of the unique patient needs from a clinical, biological, psychologic, and sociologic aspect before planning care
   c. Estimating patient expectations and building a care plan based on the patient's expressed needs so that compliance is increased
   d. All of the above
   e. None of the above

2. Oral risk assessment is based on which one of the following healthcare platforms?
   a. Health promotion
   b. Risk and risk assessment
   c. Intervention and prevention
   d. All of the above

3. The benefits of a system-based, data-gathering tool for chairside use include all *except* which one of the following?
   a. Provides a holistic approach to care
   b. Can provide for early disease intervention
   c. Provides oral risk concerns on which to build prevention strategies
   d. Predetermines insurance coding

4. To complete the assessment phase for a patient using the oral risk assessment system, which one of the following categories of information is *not* required?
   1. Health history
   2. Dental history
   3. Fluoride history
   4. Belief survey
   5. Clinical and radiographic findings
   a. *4* and *5*
   b. All except *4*
   c. *2, 3,* and *4*
   d. All elements listed are required.

5. For Ms. Wallace, the oral risk concern of gingival hyperplasia is based on which one of the following assessment tools?
   a. Clinical findings
   b. Health history
   c. Patient concern of a specific symptom
   d. All of the above

6. The evaluation of no bleeding on probing at a reevaluation appointment would be a measure of evaluation for which one of the following oral risk concerns for Ms. Wallace?
   a. Bone loss
   b. Gingival recession
   c. Gland pain
   d. Gingival hyperplasia
   e. None of the above

7. The diet survey portion of the prevention survey can provide clues in defining which oral risk concern for Ms. Wallace?
   a. Root dental caries
   b. Bone loss
   c. Trauma
   d. Gland pain

8. The terms *intervention* and *prevention* can be clearly defined; however, in dentistry, these terms often overlap.
   a. Both the statement and the clarification are true.
   b. The statement is correct; the clarification is incorrect.
   c. The statement is incorrect; the clarification is correct.
   d. Neither the statement nor the clarification is correct.

9. An example of a therapeutic intervention for Ms. Wallace would include which one of the following interventions?
   a. Fluoride treatment
   b. Debridement
   c. Diet discussion
   d. Discussion of the oral manifestations of her current medication
   e. All except *d*

10. Planning patient care is not considered a complex process because all patient care can be based on a standard, set routine.
    a. The statement is true; the rationale is false.
    b. Both the statement and the rationale are false.
    c. The statement is false; the rationale is true.
    d. Both the statement and the rationale are true.

WHERE do I go for more information or support?

evolve

For suggested web sites and agencies, additional readings and resources, and more chapter-specific information, please consult your Evolve Student Resources. Because of the ever-changing nature of the Internet, please keep in mind that web sites listed and their content may change.

 CD-ROM

Reference files: As you work through the CD-ROM exercises, you should be able to print reference files and add them to your class materials. No specific reference files apply to this chapter.

HOW can I keep track of my progress toward competence?

As an ongoing picture of progress, record and monitor clinical experiences relating to Chapter 20 content in your Portfolio.

Self-Reflection

On a regular basis, review these experiences (with a faculty member). Identify strengths, weaknesses (not just numbers), and changes that you would incorporate into your clinical care plan now that you have had these experiences.

21 Individualizing Preventive and Therapeutic Strategies

WHY do I need to know about Individualizing Preventive and Therapeutic Strategies?

The ultimate success of any dental hygiene therapy is the restoration of oral health and prevention of future disease. Engaging the patient in developing his or her own prevention strategies is challenging but also arguably the most rewarding aspect of delivering oral care (and an aspect of the profession that depends entirely on the philosophy of practice that includes the patient as a partner). This chapter details the final two steps of the oral risk assessment process, focusing on oral self-care recommendations.

WHAT will I be able to do with this knowledge?

1. State rationale for the engagement of the patient as a partner in the oral care process.
2. Compare and contrast a therapeutic intervention and a prevention strategy.
3. Explain, by way of a patient example, four logical small steps in the process of recommending products and practices for oral self-care.
4. Differentiate between a goal and a strategy.
5. Cite several obstacles to seeking dental care.
6. Discuss components important to consider in planning oral care.
7. Defend the value of evaluation and reevaluation as a way of ensuring optimal oral health.
8. Map a patient's care plan in therapeutic intervention, prevention, and evaluation and reevaluation.
9. Apply Steps 4 and 5 of the oral risk assessment process to any patient.
10. Recognize the value of a systematized holistic approach to oral care.

HOW do I prepare myself to transfer this knowledge to patient care?

 Go to Chapter 21 content on your CD-ROM or search for "Oral Risk Assessment."

CD Exercises

- *21-1 to 21-9: Step 5: Reevaluation:* Following a narrated and animated demonstration of the oral risk assessment process, complete any or all patient assessments as desired or assigned.

Textbook

Review Case Study 21-1, Individualizing Prevention Strategies, and the case applications. After reading the applications, consider the following additional questions:
- Based on your knowledge of patient and human behavior, do you think that the outcome of prevention discussions with Ms. Wallace will be positive?
- What if Ms. Wallace did not believe prevention of oral problems was important?
- Would you address her needs differently?
- What if she believed that she was unable to make any changes in personal habits at this time? Would your course of action and or patient goals change?

HOW do I perform these skills?

evolve

A printable version of this checklist is available on your Evolve Student Resources.
To design successful clinical therapy and appropriate personalized patient care, I will:
- ☐ Review all of the patient's records.
- ☐ Analyze oral risk concerns.
- ☐ Plan therapeutic intervention and prevention strategies.
- ☐ Recommend personalized oral self-care products and practices.
- ☐ Reevaluate all outcomes.

HOW can I more effectively use this knowledge?

Critical Thinking Activities

Use the following worksheet to complete your activities.
1. Together with a classmate, in a role-playing format, perform Steps 1, 2, 3, and 4 of the oral risk assessment worksheet. Were there any pertinent findings from this step that you previously overlooked? Did any biological, psychologic, or sociologic elements come to light that might be used in planning prevention strategies?
2. Make a list of as many prevention strategies as you can. Determine whether each acts strictly as a prevention strategy, as a therapeutic intervention, or as both.

103

3. Using Worksheet #1, perform Steps 4 and 5 on a student partner. What types of patient goals and prevention strategies can you document?
4. Select a student from the second-year class. Present different clinical outcomes and ask which supportive care steps he or she would recommend.
5. If you are a first-year student, select a second-year student with whom to work. Ask to review the dental records of a patient he or she is currently treating. After completing Steps 1, 2, and 3 of the oral risk assessment worksheet with the use of only the dental records provided, complete Steps 4 and 5. Determine the clinical goal, therapeutic intervention, patient goal, prevention strategy, and evaluation method for each oral risk concern noted. Would this process have been more thorough with a prevention survey?

Worksheet #1—Oral Risk Assessment Worksheet

Patient Name _____   Date _____

I

REVIEW		
Health History	**Medications & Dose**	**Duration**
❑ Cardiovascular (heart)	(prescription and OTC)	
❑ Central nervous system (nerves)		
❑ Endocrine (endocrine glands)		
❑ Gastrointestinal (stomach, intestines)		
❑ Genitourinary (sex organs, urinary tract)		
❑ Head, eyes, ears, nose, throat		
❑ Hematologic (blood)		
❑ Integumentary (skin)		
❑ Musculoskeletal (muscles, bones, joints)		
❑ Psychologic		
❑ Respiratory		

Vital Signs BP   /   Pulse

Dental History

❑ Sensitive teeth	❑ Sore jaw	❑ Toothache	❑ Sore gums	❑ Clenching
❑ Bleeding gums	❑ Difficulty chewing	❑ Filling fell out	❑ Dry mouth	❑ Grinding
❑ Bad breath	❑ Burning sensation		❑ Abscess	❑ Swollen face
❑ Swelling inside mouth	❑ Tartar buildup	❑ Yellowing teeth	❑ Difficulty swallowing	
❑ Adequate OH time	❑ Anxiety/Pain	❑ Oral self-care difficulty		

Oral Health Products:

Fluoride History

❑ Fluoridated water	❑ Away from home >4 days/week	❑ Oral rinse w/fluoride	
❑ Water filter	❑ Bottled juice	Child:	
❑ Bottled water	❑ Fluoridated dentifrice	❑ In daycare w/out fluoride	❑ Supplements

Behaviors

❑ Annual physical	❑ Balance work/relaxation	❑ Tobacco use	❑ Exercise
❑ Follows medical advice	❑ Eating habits controlled	❑ Alcohol use	
❑ Follows dental advice	❑ Increased stress	❑ Caffeine use	

Diet Survey   ❑ Carbohydrate/Sucrose intake (excessive/moderate/minimal)

Beliefs

❑ Understands oral status	❑ Values prevention
❑ Wants product recommendations	❑ Open to change ❑ Feels in control of oral condition

Clinical and Radiographic Findings

Intraoral/Extraoral Examination	❑ Within normal limits		❑ See chart
Caries	❑ Coronal	❑ Interproximal	❑ Root surface

Restorations/Prosthetics

Restorations	❑ Amalgam	❑ Composite	❑ Crowns/inlays/onlays	❑ Bridges
Dentures	❑ Complete	❑ Partial		

Periodontium

❑ Recession	❑ Plaque ❑ Bleeding on probing	❑ Loss of attached gingiva	❑ Pockets <3mm
❑ Mucogingival defects			

Occlusion/TMJ	❑ Traumatic occlusion	❑ Crepitus	
Bone Loss	❑ <25%	❑ 25-50%	❑ Horizontal	❑ Vertical

Continued

Chapter **21** **Individualizing Preventive and Therapeutic Strategies**

II

ANALYZE
Oral Risk Concerns

At risk for   Clinically Evident

Hard Tissues

- ❑ Abrasion/Attrition/Erosion   ❑
- ❑ Bone Loss   ❑
- ❑ Bruxism/Occlusal Trauma   ❑
- ❑ Calculus   ❑
- ❑ Caries: coronal/interproximal   ❑
- ❑ Caries: root surface   ❑
- ❑ Chipped broken teeth   ❑
- ❑ Extrinsic staining   ❑
- ❑ Fluorosis   ❑
- ❑ Intrinsic staining   ❑
- ❑ Malaligned teeth   ❑
- ❑ Mobile teeth   ❑
- ❑ Sensitive teeth   ❑
- ❑ Trauma   ❑
- ❑ Other   ❑

Soft Tissues

- ❑ Abscess: carious   ❑
- ❑ Abscess: periodontal   ❑
- ❑ Atrophic ulcer   ❑
- ❑ Aphthous ulcer   ❑
- ❑ Burning tongue/mouth   ❑
- ❑ Candidiasis   ❑
- ❑ Ecchymosis   ❑
- ❑ Gingival recession   ❑
- ❑ Gingival hyperplasia   ❑
- ❑ Gingivitis   ❑
- ❑ Herpetic lesions   ❑
- ❑ Increased plaque   ❑
- ❑ Leukoplakia   ❑
- ❑ Lichen planus   ❑
- ❑ Oral cancer   ❑
- ❑ Periodontal disease   ❑
- ❑ Petechiae   ❑
- ❑ Salivation – increased   ❑
- ❑ Salivation – decreased   ❑
- ❑ Trauma   ❑
- ❑ Xerostomia   ❑
- ❑ Other_____   ❑

Consult   Referral

- ❑ Consultation with physician   ❑
- ❑ Consultation with dental specialist   ❑

III

PLAN		
Clinical Goals	**Therapeutic Intervention**	**Patient Goals**

Continued

IV

V

ORAL CARE RECOMMENDATIONS		EVALUATE
Prevention Strategy	**Toothbrush** **Product**	**Clinical Goals**
	❑ Mechanical	
	❑ Child ❑ Youth ❑ Compact ❑ Full	
	❑ Soft ❑ Extra Soft	
	❑ Powered	
	Brushing frequency	
	Brushing duration	
	Interdental Cleaning Products	
	❑ Floss Type Frequency	
	❑ Oral Irrigator Frequency	
	❑ Interdental Brush Frequency	
	❑ Other	
	Dentifrice	
	❑ Fluoride ❑ Whitening	
	❑ Sensitivity ❑ Multiple Benefit	
	❑ Tartar Control ❑ Gingival Benefit	
	❑ Children's	
	Oral Rinse	
	❑ Fluoride	
	❑ Cosmetic	**Patient Goals**
	❑ Alcohol-free	
	❑ Tartar Control	
	❑ Chlorhexidine	
	❑ Essential Oil/Phenol Compound	
	Prosthodontic Care	
	❑ Adhesive ❑ Denture Brush	
	❑ Denture Bath/Cleanser	
	Self Evaluation	
	❑ Disclosing tablets or solutions	
	❑ Evaluate bleeding points	
	Other	

DO I have all the answers?

Review Questions

Check your answers against the Answer Key at the back of this Study Guide to assess what you have learned. Questions 4 to 6, 8, and 10 refer to Case Study 21-1.

1. Which one of the following characterizes the act of personalizing patient oral self-care instructions?
   a. Important to engage the patient as a partner
   b. Part of patient-centered treatment philosophy
   c. Helpful to the dental hygienist in terms of job satisfaction
   d. *a* and *b* only
   e. All of the above

2. Which step in the oral risk assessment system *recommends* oral self-care products and practices?
   a. Step 1
   b. Step 3
   c. Step 4
   d. Step 2
   e. Step 5

3. Reevaluation of supportive care includes which one of the following?
   a. Only the debrided portion of the treatment plan
   b. Patient compliance
   c. Dental caries rate
   d. Review all aspects of supportive care process, including both therapeutic intervention and prevention strategies

4. Oral risk concerns for Ms. Wallace include all of the following *except* which one?
   a. Increase in plaque
   b. Lichen planus
   c. Gingival hyperplasia
   d. Tooth mobility
   e. *a* and *c* only

5. Of the prevention strategies for Ms. Wallace, which one of the following addresses the oral risk concern for gingival hyperplasia?
   a. Discussion of host defense mechanisms
   b. Discussion and plan of supportive care appointments
   c. Discussion of role of saliva in remineralization process
   d. Discussion of possible oral effects of her current medications
   e. None of the above

6. Which one of the following obstacles to care should be considered in the planning of supportive care appointments for Ms. Wallace?
   a. Transportation
   b. Confusion about dental terminology
   c. Illiteracy
   d. Poor perception of dentistry
   e. None of the above

7. In determining the appropriate appointment sequencing, which one of the following should be followed as a goal of therapy?
   a. Remove gross debris only at the first appointment so that the patient's tolerance will increase with time.
   b. Complete therapy that is initiated.
   c. Always begin on anterior teeth so that the patient can see a difference.
   d. Follow the wishes of the patient.

8. Which reevaluation measure or measures are appropriate for Ms. Wallace in determining whether she has met the goal of understanding signs and symptoms of gingival disease?
   a. She can pick out a photo of diseased gingiva.
   b. She can point to any areas in her mouth that she feels are not responding to therapy.
   c. She can point out areas in her mouth that require polishing.
   d. She can cite the symptoms of gingival inflammation.
   e. *a*, *b*, and *d* only

9. The five steps in the oral risk assessment system include all *except* which one of the following?
   a. Carefully reviewing all patient data
   b. Determining oral risk concerns
   c. Mapping each appointment
   d. Evaluating therapy
   e. Evaluating clinician satisfaction

10. Of the following factors for Ms. Wallace, which are the most important factors to address in helping provide her with a future of optimal oral health?
    1. Lack of oral self-care tools
    2. Not understanding the oral effects of prescription medication
    3. Not seeking regular dental care
    4. Lack of appreciation for her role in disease prevention
    5. Not spending adequate time on oral self-care
    a. *1* and *3*
    b. *1*, *4*, and *5*
    c. *2* and *3*
    d. All of the above
    e. None of the above

WHERE do I go for more information or support?

 evolve

For suggested web sites and agencies, additional readings and resources, and more chapter-specific information, please consult your Evolve Student Resources. Because of the ever-changing nature of the Internet, please keep in mind that web sites listed and their content may change.

CD-ROM

Reference files: As you work through the CD-ROM exercises, you should be able to print reference files and add them to your class materials. No specific reference files apply to this chapter.

HOW can I keep track of my progress toward competence?

As an ongoing picture of progress, record and monitor clinical experiences relating to Chapter 21 content in your Portfolio.

Self-Reflection

On a regular basis, review these experiences (with a faculty member). Identify strengths, weaknesses (not just numbers), and changes that you would incorporate into your clinical care plan now that you have had these experiences.

22 Posttreatment Assessment and Supportive Care

WHY do I need to know about Posttreatment Assessment and Supportive Care?

The dental hygienist will treat a variety of patients who have periodontal conditions and other chronic oral ailments. Tailoring treatment to the specific needs of the patient is the first step toward improving and maintaining health. Periodontal maintenance (PM) and supportive care appointments designed with the patient's needs in mind are an essential part of dental hygiene practice.

WHAT will I be able to do with this knowledge?

1. Identify patients whose oral health risks and problems require close intervals for supportive care or continuation of care for other oral problems.
2. Recognize symptoms or conditions that indicate referral or co-management with the periodontist and discuss them with the patient.
3. Plan a supportive care program based on the patient's disease control skills and the risk of disease recurrence.
4. Identify successful or reasonable outcomes, which may vary from patient to patient.
5. Document everything.
6. Evaluate current literature on the topic of supportive care intervals.

HOW do I prepare myself to transfer this knowledge to patient care?

 Go to Chapter 22 content on your CD-ROM or search for "Periodontal Disease" or "Dental Caries."

CD Exercises

- *22-1: Risk Assessment—Ann Cronin, George Burkett, William Johnston, Maria Bjork, Eva Bjork, Terrence Zellar, Subra Mani, Elena Guri, Adolfo Santana:* Identify patient risk factors for periodontal disease.
- *22-2: Risk Assessment:* Based on patient records from the patient family, identify periodontal risk factors.
- *22-3: Dental Caries:* Identify factors that place a patient at risk for dental caries.
- *22-4: Dental Caries—Ann Cronin, George Burkett, William Johnston, Maria Bjork, Eva Bjork, Terrence Zellar, Subra Mani, Elena Guri, Adolfo Santana:* Based on patient records from the patient family, identify dental caries risk factors.

Textbook

Review Case Study 22-1, Evaluating Periodontal Outcomes, and the case applications. After reading the chapter, consider the following questions:

- What is the patient's risk level for recurrence of the disease?
- What are the patient's attitude and psychomotor abilities in controlling the disease?
- Which kinds of supportive-care procedures are best for different patients?
- Based on the patient's primary problem, what is the optimal interval length for supportive care?

HOW do I perform these skills?

evolve

A printable version of this checklist is available on your Evolve Student Resources.

To evaluate the continuation of supportive care, I will:

- ☐ Create a prevention program.
- ☐ Determine patients' needs, problems, and general health status.
- ☐ Identify the intended outcomes.
  - ☐ Periodontal reevaluation:
    - ☐ Review patient records and radiographs.
    - ☐ Update health history.
    - ☐ Listen to patient's comments, observations, or concerns.
    - ☐ Perform head and neck examination.
    - ☐ Perform a hard tissue examination.
  - ☐ Periodontal examination:
    - ☐ Review patient's personal care, behaviors, and attitudes.
    - ☐ Perform debridement as necessary.
    - ☐ Perform polishing as needed.
    - ☐ Schedule subsequent supportive care appointments.
  - ☐ Dental caries reevaluation:
    - ☐ Review patient records and radiographs.
    - ☐ Update health history.
    - ☐ Listen to patient's comments, observations, and concerns.
    - ☐ Perform head and neck examination.
    - ☐ Perform a hard tissue examination.
    - ☐ Evaluate dental caries status.

□ Review patient's personal care, behaviors, and attitudes.

□ Apply topical fluoride, if appropriate.

□ Schedule subsequent supportive care appointments.

HOW can I more effectively use this knowledge?

Critical Thinking Activities

Use the following worksheet to complete activity #1.

1. With the emphasis on evidence-based care, some of the same questions regarding the interval of patient care must be periodically reexamined. Search the dental literature for the answers to the following questions:

   a. Is 3 months still the recommended interval for supportive care for patients with periodontitis?

   b. What are the desired outcomes of successful periodontal maintenance (PM)?

   c. How should supportive periodontal care (SPC) outcomes be determined: clinically, microbially, through diagnostic testing, or by laboratory analyses?

   d. What are the parameters for each type of SPC outcome?

   e. According to the dental literature on evidence-based care, what are the current recommendations on the use of pharmacotherapeutic agents and controlled delivery as adjunctive antimicrobial/antibiotic therapies?

2. Find the report of the 1994 1st European Workshop on Periodontology and study the concept of SPC as described in this workshop. What are the parallel descriptions or terms used by the American Academy of Periodontology? Refer to the association's web site and read the position paper and parameters of care for maintenance therapy.

3. For periodontal patients whom you see for more than one appoinment, keep a journal of what appears to motivate each patient. Write down whether patient observations were helpful (or not helpful). Examine your notes to determine whether anything appears to be aiding concordance for different patients. Could some aspect of the patient's attitude or some behavior on your part encourage the patient to improve plaque control and adhere to the appropriate interval of care?

4. Role-play the part of a dental hygienist faced with a pleasant but nonconcordant patient. Develop the skills of listening to the patient's difficulties, such as plaque control, keeping appointments, finances, time, or dealing with more than one office. Practice responding to patient concerns in a beneficial and positive manner. (Hint for patient role-player: Mention any and all problems, reasons, and excuses you can think of for why you are not responsible for conditions in your mouth.)

Worksheet #1
Record your findings from Critical Thinking Activity #1 on this worksheet.

OVERVIEW
Article title _____

Authors _____

Publication title _____

Date, volume, issue, and page _____

Stated purpose of the study _____

What was being evaluated? _____

METHODOLOGY
Study Design
Was the study design clearly described
and appropriate for the investigation? _____

Was the study design double blinded? _____

Was the study design single blinded? _____

Was the length of investigation sufficient
to study the subject? _____

Was interexaminer and intraexaminer
reliability stated? _____

Subjects
Was the sample size large enough? _____

Composition of the sample population:
Was it appropriate to the therapy used? _____

How many subjects dropped out of the study
(through attrition)? _____

Did the researchers attempt to balance the
groups? _____

Product Usage
Supervised? _____

Special protocol? _____

Ad lib? _____

Was it the same for both the control and the
experimental group?

Continued

Chapter **22** **Posttreatment Assessment and Supportive Care**

DATA ANALYSIS

By what methods will the data be analyzed? _____

What statistical methods were to be used? _____

At what value was the statistical
significance set? $P =$ _____

RESULTS

Were all groups reported? _____

Were the results statistically significant? _____

DISCUSSIONS, SUMMARY, CONCLUSION

Was the clinical significance part of the
discussion? _____

Was the statistical information enough to
verify the results? _____

Did the discussions and concluding
statements relate appropriately to the
stated purpose of the study? _____

Did the author demonstrate a scientific basis
for the recommendation of a new agent,
product, or therapy? _____

Were limitations of the study discussed? _____

Was the research question answered? _____

Did the author or authors call for further
research? _____

DO I have all the answers?

Review Questions

Check your answers against the Answer Key at the back of this Study Guide to assess what you have learned.
The following questions refer to Case Study 22-1.

1. Mrs. Lightfoot is taking prescription drugs for her medical problems. For which illness might she be taking medication that could have an adverse effect on her plaque biofilm control?
   a. Non–insulin-dependent diabetes mellitus (NIDDM)
   b. High blood pressure
   c. Osteoarthritis
   d. Congestive heart failure (CHF)

2. Which of the following would be the least likely reason for the increased bleeding Mrs. Lightfoot shows?
   a. Gingival hyperplasia
   b. Hyperglycemia
   c. Poor plaque biofilm control
   d. A change in the diuretic prescribed

3. In Mrs. Lightfoot's case, which of the following is the most likely reason her probe measurements are greater?
   a. Poor probe technique
   b. An increase in gingival margin height
   c. Apical migration of periodontal attachment
   d. Poor plaque biofilm control

4. Based on the information you have on Mrs. Lightfoot, how would you schedule her next SPC session?
   a. Schedule her appointment in 2 months.
   b. Recommend that she visit a dental hygienist while she is traveling.
   c. Schedule her next SPC appointment for when she returns from her trip.
   d. Wait until she returns from her trip to schedule her appointment.

5. Which of the following do you think is the most serious problem Mrs. Lightfoot faces?
   a. She will be unable to keep her 3-month appointment interval.
   b. Her plaque biofilm control is poor.
   c. Her bleeding index is now 25%.
   d. She does not understand her role in controlling periodontal disease.

6. Which of the following illnesses might hamper Mrs. Lightfoot's ability to remove plaque from her teeth?
   a. NIDDM
   b. High blood pressure
   c. Osteoarthritis
   d. CHF

WHERE do I go for more information or support?

evolve

For suggested web sites and agencies, additional readings and resources, and more chapter-specific information, please consult your Evolve Student Resources. Because of the ever-changing nature of the Internet, please keep in mind that web sites listed and their content may change.

CD-ROM

Reference files: As you work through the CD-ROM exercises, you should be able to print reference files and add them to your class materials. No specific reference files apply to this chapter.

HOW can I keep track of my progress toward competence?

As an ongoing picture of progress, record and monitor clinical experiences relating to Chapter 22 content in your Portfolio.

Self-Reflection

On a regular basis, review these experiences (with a faculty member). Identify strengths, weaknesses (not just numbers), and changes that you would incorporate into your clinical care plan now that you have had these experiences.

23 Case Development, Documentation, and Presentation

WHY do I need to know about Case Development, Documentation, and Presentation?

The clinical dental hygienist works with various cases throughout the work day. Case development and documentation exercises provide the framework of information necessary for complex decision making and treatment recommendations for individual patient's needs and clinical situations. Developed cases can then be presented in various forms to promote learning and professional development.

WHAT will I be able to do with this knowledge?

1. Provide an example of how case development and documentation may be used.
2. Analyze the purpose, the intended audience, and the goal of case development in a given situation.
3. Identify the components that can be developed and documented on a given case.
4. Compile all material necessary to document the therapeutic interventions and strategies of patient care provided in the case being developed.
5. Demonstrate case presentation skills to peers and other professionals in either written or oral format.

HOW do I prepare myself to transfer this knowledge to patient care?

 Go to Chapter 23 content on your CD-ROM or search for "Case Development."

CD Exercises

- *23-1: Summary of Case Development, Documentation and Presentation:* Look at topics given, and then select the most appropriate candidate from the patient family.
- *23-2: Case Development and Documentation Assignment:* Look at the patient family, and then determine the topics that might be developed into a case presentation.
- *23-3: Case Documentation Guidelines:* Look at various case elements in a form from which you can complete a patient case topic of your own selection for faculty review and feedback.

Textbook

Review Case Study 23-1, Use of Patient Case Documentation for Extended Learning, and the case applications.

HOW do I perform these skills?

evolve

A printable version of this checklist is available on your Evolve Student Resources.
To develop, document, and present a case, I will:
- ☐ Define purpose.
- ☐ Define audience.
- ☐ Define topic.
- ☐ Document patient information.
- ☐ Document demographic and health history assessment.
- ☐ Document clinical assessment.
- ☐ Document strategies in therapy and patient instruction.
- ☐ Document actual therapeutic and preventive care of the patient.
- ☐ Provide visual representation of the patient's clinical findings.
- ☐ Provide study questions and answers.
- ☐ Describe posttherapy clinical evaluation findings of the patient.
- ☐ Present case to intended audience.

HOW can I more effectively use this knowledge?

Case representation of patient care can be used in several ways. The first and perhaps most obvious is patient education. The statement *a picture is worth a thousand words* is true when motivating a person to change oral care behavior or encouraging a patient to continue the present course. Documenting the changes or progression of health may motivate the patient and the dental hygienist.

Critical Thinking Activities

Use the following worksheet to complete activity #1.
1. From your family of patients, identify those with oral and systemic diseases whose condition would warrant documentation. Select an audience for the presentation of your documentation.
2. Role-play with a peer the discussion you would have with a patient to request permission to document his or her case.

Worksheet #1

Use this form to develop a case study on one of your clinic patients, or use one of the patients from the CD-ROM.

Purpose (State the reason for presenting the case.) _____

_____

_____

Audience (Define the audience for the presentation.) _____

_____

_____

Selection criteria (State the criteria by which you selected the case for presentation.) _____

_____

_____

Patient Information

Profile (Summary of the basic information about the patient) _____

_____

_____

Chief concern (Summary of the main reason for patient visit) _____

_____

_____

Health history (Summary of health-related findings) _____

_____

_____

Medical or dental indications (Summary of significant dental or medical instructions with medications or health systems) _____

_____

_____

Clinical Assessment

Extraoral examination (Summarization) _____

_____

_____

Intraoral examination (Summarization) _____

_____

_____

Current dental condition (Summarization) _____

_____

_____

Radiographic examination (Summarization) _____

_____

_____

Periodic examination (Summarization) _____

_____

_____

Continued

119

Worksheet #1—cont'd

Oral risk assessment (Summarization)

_____
_____

Current oral self-care routine (Summarization)

_____
_____
_____
_____

Referral needs (Summarization)

_____
_____
_____

Planning Phase

Rationale for case selection (Summarization)

_____
_____
_____

Treatment goals and outcomes (Summarization)

_____
_____
_____

Initial therapeutic strategies (Summarization)

_____
_____
_____

Preventive educational strategy (Summarization)

_____
_____
_____

Instrumentation strategy (Summarization)

_____
_____
_____

Discussion points

_____
_____
_____

Consent signed

_____
_____
_____

Implementation Phase

Appointments

_____
_____
_____

Services completed

_____
_____
_____

Chapter **23**   **Case Development, Documentation, and Presentation**

Worksheet #1—cont'd

Treatment revisions

_____
_____
_____

Patient care

_____
_____
_____

Self-care

_____
_____
_____
_____

Case Assets (Checklist)

☐ Intraoral photographs
☐ Study models
☐ Radiographs
☐ Dental charting
☐ Diet survey
☐ Periodontal charting
☐ Oral risk assessment

Continued

Worksheet #1—cont'd
Study Questions

Questions   Answers

1. _____   _____

2. _____   _____

Posttreatment Evaluation

Intraoral photographs (Take as indicated.)   _____

_____

_____

Chief complaint (Review whether completed care   _____
addressed goals, risks, patient concerns: summary of
health history update and changes in the intraoral and   _____
extraoral examinations.)
_____

Periodontal examination (Summary of probe depths,   _____
bleeding on probing, plaque biofilm index, and gingival
description.)   _____

_____

Oral self-care outcomes (Summary of patient's   _____
understanding and effectiveness of oral hygiene, current
recommendations based on indices (e.g., bleeding index   _____
[BI], plaque biofilm index [PI], bleeding on probing
[BOP], and gingival description.)   _____

Therapeutic outcomes (Summary of effectiveness of   _____
previously performed periodontal therapy and assessment
of patient response.)   _____

_____

Discussion points   _____

_____

_____

Future care recommendations   _____

_____

_____

Referrals (Specify protocol.)   _____

_____

_____

Active therapy (Possible need for further therapy.)   _____

_____

_____

Worksheet #1—cont'd

Supportive-care interval (Interval recommendation for
follow-up care.)

_____

_____

_____

**Student Evaluation of Therapeutic and
Preventive Outcomes**

Summarize key concepts from the case presentation.

_____

_____

_____

_____

List the modifications that would enhance treatment
outcomes.

_____

_____

_____

_____

_____

Chapter **23** **Case Development, Documentation, and Presentation**

DO I have all the answers?

Review Questions

Check your answers against the Answer Key at the back of this Study Guide to assess what you have learned.

1. Which of the following is(are) example(s) of how a case documentation and presentation can be used?
   a. Education of peers and patients
   b. Patient education and motivation
   c. Third-party payer reimbursement
   d. Evaluation of the outcome of care
   e. All of the above
2. Which one of the following must be considered before a case is developed?
   a. Age of patient
   b. Intended audience
   c. Medical history
   d. All of the above
3. Which one of the following is a part of the patient profile section of case development?
   a. Complete radiographic series
   b. Treatment strategies
   c. Current and historical dental information
   d. Initial clinical assessment
   e. Extraoral and intraoral examination (EIX)
4. Which one of the following presentation formats are the most widely used?
   a. Written
   b. Oral
   c. Electronic
   d. All of the above

WHERE do I go for more information or support?

evolve

For suggested web sites and agencies, additional readings and resources, and more chapter-specific information, please consult your Evolve Student Resources. Because of the ever-changing nature of the Internet, please keep in mind that web sites listed and their content may change.

 CD-ROM

Reference files: As you work through the CD-ROM exercises, you should be able to print reference files and add them to your class materials. No specific reference files apply to this chapter.

HOW can I keep track of my progress toward competence?

As an ongoing picture of progress, record and monitor clinical experiences relating to Chapter 23 content in your Portfolio.

Self-Reflection

On a regular basis, review these experiences (with a faculty member). Identify strengths, weaknesses (not just numbers), and changes that you would incorporate into your clinical care plan now that you have had these experiences.

24 Devices for Oral Self-Care

WHY do I need to know about Devices for Oral Self-Care?

Dental plaque biofilm control is the most important factor in obtaining and sustaining optimal oral health. Plaque (i.e., dental biofilm) must be mechanically removed, and daily cleaning with a toothbrush and other interdental aids is the most dependable means by which to achieve and maintain this status. The role and professional responsibility of a dental hygienist is to provide oral health education and skill development for each patient as part of comprehensive dental hygiene patient care. Importantly, oral hygiene instruction for plaque biofilm control should be patient centered and individualized to meet the patient's oral conditions and biopsychosocial aspects and abilities to ensure optimal adherence to an oral self-care regimen.

WHAT will I be able to do with this knowledge?

1. Describe and explain the appropriate use of and oral health indications for the following categories of oral self-care devices: toothbrushes, interdental cleaners, dental floss, and dental water jet.
2. Identify the appropriate components of a randomized clinical trial.
3. Provide a rationale for oral self-care product selection based on evidence-based decision making, patient need, and anatomical considerations.
4. Explain the role of self-evaluation in plaque biofilm control. Explain how disclosing solutions or tablets can be used in a patient's individualized oral self-care plan.
5. Monitor and recommend modifications for patient use of oral self-care products based on therapeutic intervention planning.
6. Provide a rationale for recommending a manual or powered toothbrush to a patient.
7. Describe features that can be found on modern powered toothbrushes.
8. Identify differences in the mechanism of action among different types of powered toothbrushes.
9. Demonstrate the appropriate way to use the jet tip, irrigator tip, and the Pik Pocket tip to a patient.
10. Determine the appropriate irrigation tip to recommend to a patient.

HOW do I prepare myself to transfer this knowledge to patient care?

CD *Go to Chapter 24 content on your CD-ROM or search for "Toothbrushes," "Interproximal Cleaning," or "Oral Irrigation."*

CD Exercises

- *24-1: Manual Toothbrush:* Match the correct terminology to the characteristics of the handle, head, and bristle design.
- *24-2: Power Brushes:* Identify different modalities of powered toothbrushes.
- *24-3: Toothbrushing Techniques:* Identify the brushing methods from video.
- *24-4: Toothbrushing Techniques:* Match the intraoral condition to the most appropriate brushing method.
- *24-5: Interdental Cleaning—Reference File:* Match the purpose, instructions for use, and precautions to interproximal cleaning devices; then write the exercise to the reference file.
- *24-6 to 24-9: Interdental Cleaning:* Recommend interdental cleaning based on need for patients Ann Cronin, Eva Bjork, Terrance Zellar, and Adolfo Santana.
- *24-10: Dental Water Jet—Ann Cronin:* Identify the proper way to use a home irrigation device for Ann Cronin.

Textbook

Review Case Study 24-1, Specific Oral Self-Care Recommendations, and the case applications. After reading the chapter, consider the following questions:

- Will Mrs. Cronin's lips be elastic enough to get a cleaning device to the distal of the maxillary second molars with ease?
- How much room exists between the cheeks and the gingival one third of the tooth?
- How can Mrs. Cronin be guided to clean the gingival margins more effectively?
- What questions would you have regarding tooth positions, recession, clefting, rolled margins, and interproximal embrasure spaces?

For important concepts and application of knowledge, review tables, figures, and boxed sections of the book.

The following chapter elements may be especially helpful for clinical transfer and may be used as a clinical reference:

- Table 24-1: CONSORT Checklist and Flowchart Guidelines for Improving the Reporting of Clinical Trials
- Table 24-2: Toothbrushing Methods
- Table 24-3: Interdental Aids for Embrasure Types
- Box 24-4: Patient Factors to Consider When Making Oral Self-Care Recommendations

HOW can I more effectively use this knowledge?

Critical Thinking Activities

Use the following worksheet to complete activity #1.

1. Interview or survey four individuals regarding their oral self-care activities. Record and summarize the findings, and discuss the expected and unexpected results.
   a. Evaluate the design of each toothbrush (head and handle shape, bristle configuration and type, and wear). How many need replacing?
   b. Determine the number of times each individual brushes per day and the average length of time each spends on brushing.
   c. Determine how and when each individual uses interdental cleaning products.
   d. Inquire as to the method each individual uses for self-assessment of plaque removal.
   e. Record the oral care instructions received from the oral healthcare provider. Determine which dental professional gave the instructions.
2. Evaluate five patient charts for the type of dental cleaning recommendations given. Summarize the results and discuss the expected and unexpected results.
3. Select the appropriate irrigation tip and use an oral irrigator in your own mouth.
4. Select a patient with periodontal probe depths (PDs) of less than 4 mm. Take preirrigation and postirrigation samples to examine under the microscope. Keep preirrigation and postirrigation bleeding indices over a period of time. Do the same for each controlled-delivery system used.
5. Select one irrigation tip or one chemotherapeutic agent to research in-depth and report to your class.

Worksheet #1

Use this worksheet with Critical Thinking Activity #1.

Interview or survey four individuals (friends, family, colleagues) regarding oral self-care products and habits. Use the following form to collect the data and respond to the accompanying questions.

1. Evaluate the design of each of their toothbrushes (handle and head shape, bristle configuration, and wear). Do any need replacing?

	Person 1	Person 2	Person 3	Person 4
Toothbrush design Head type				
Bristle type				
Handle type				
Last replacement (number of months)				
Length of brushing time				
Interdental cleaning aids				
Floss				
Toothpick				
Other				
None				
What methods are used to determine oral cleanliness?				
On what do they base their product selection?				
Any unmet oral hygiene needs?				

2. Evaluate just the toothbrush replacement interval for each patient. Is it appropriate? What information would you give to influence a change in their behavior?

	Patient 1	Person 2	Patient 3	Patient 4
Interval:				
Appropriate?				
Behavior modification:				

Continued

127

3. What is an average length of brushing time? Is it appropriate? What types of changes would you suggest based on just this knowledge?

	Patient 1	Patient 2	Patient 3	Patient 4
Brushing time:				
Appropriate?				
Behavior modification:				

4. What methods are reported to determine oral cleanliness? What additional suggestions would you offer?

	Patient 1	Patient 2	Patient 3	Patient 4
Self-assessment method to determine plaque biofilm removal:				
Appropriate?				
Behavior modification:				

5. On what does each patient seem to base product selection? What changes might you suggest?

	Patient 1	Patient 2	Patient 3	Patient 4
Product selection basis:				
Appropriate?				
Behavior modification:				

6. Did the patient report any unmet oral hygiene needs? If yes, then what recommendations would you have for each?

	Patient 1	Patient 2	Patient 3	Patient 4
Unmet oral hygiene need:				
Suggestion:				

DO I have all the answers?

Review Questions

Check your answers against the Answer Key at the back of this Study Guide to assess what you have learned. All questions refer to Case Study 24-1.

1. Which of the following may result from the use of a stiffer toothbrush than Mrs. Cronin was using?
   a. Ineffective plaque removal
   b. Dentinal abrasion
   c. Dentin sensitivity
   d. Excessive wear on brush
   e. All of the above

2. Mrs. Cronin cannot take her powered toothbrush on vacation. Which of the following toothbrushes would you recommend she purchase?
   a. Large handle, multitufted small head
   b. Regular handle, flat-bristle medium head
   c. Child-size toothbrush
   d. Large handle, multitufted large head

3. Which of the following brushing methods should you teach Mrs. Cronin to use with her manual toothbrush while on vacation?
   a. Modified Bass method
   b. Fones method
   c. Charters method
   d. Scrub brush method

4. All of the following are advantages for Mrs. Cronin in the use of the ultrafine interproximal brush *except* which one?
   a. Easy to use
   b. Adapts well to the proximal surface
   c. Adapts well to the facial and palatal and lingual surface
   d. Adapts well to the subgingival surface

5. Respond to Mrs. Cronin's question, "My sister loves to use waxed dental floss, but she heard that unwaxed floss is better. What do you think?"
   a. "Both work well. She should use the floss that is easiest for her."
   b. "Unwaxed is better because this type of floss is easier to use."
   c. "Unwaxed is better because this type of floss is thinner."
   d. "Waxed floss leaves a wax residue, so do not use it."

6. Mrs. Cronin has asked, "How frequently should I replace the head on my powered toothbrush?" How do you respond?
   a. "Every 3 months."
   b. "When the brush begins to show wear."
   c. "After you have been ill, especially after a cold."
   d. All of the above.

7. Mrs. Cronin's 12-year-old granddaughter has normal gingival tissue, tight contacts, and several rotated teeth. Which of the following interdental aids is the best recommendation for her?
   a. Unwaxed floss
   b. Waxed floss
   c. Proximal brush
   d. Triangular wood stick

8. Mrs. Cronin's son-in-law just purchased a natural bristle toothbrush. Which of the following bristle types would you recommend as a replacement?
   a. Soft, natural bristle
   b. Medium, natural bristle
   c. Soft, nylon bristle
   d. Medium, nylon bristle

9. After Mrs. Cronin brushes, she uses a disclosing solution to check her plaque control. She reports that she notices a thin area of plaque remaining at the gingival margin. Which of the following recommendations should be made?
   a. Use an interproximal brush.
   b. Use waxed floss.
   c. Brush for a longer period of time.
   d. Angle the head of the toothbrush so that the initial placement is against the gingiva at the gingival one third of the tooth.

10. Which of the following is the best response to Mrs. Cronin when she requests a recommendation to more effectively brush her disabled neighbor's teeth?
    a. Use a small brush head with circular strokes.
    b. Use a multiangle brush head with the modified Stillman's method.
    c. Use a powered brush with a scrub technique.
    d. Use a powered brush guided slowly and gently around the mouth.

11. Which of the following brushing methods is best recommended for Mrs. Cronin's 6-year-old grandson?
    a. Scrub brush method
    b. Fones method
    c. Modified Bass method
    d. Rolling-stroke method

12. Living with her daughter and family, Mrs. Cronin has had the opportunity to observe her grandchildren's toothbrushing habits. She reports, "My grandchildren scrub their teeth much too quickly. How long should they be brushing?" How would you respond?
    a. "Thirty to 45 seconds seems to be the average for kids."
    b. "One minute is advised."
    c. "Three minutes will get the job done."
    d. "Five minutes."

13. Respond to Mrs. Cronin's question: "Do stiffer bristles achieve better oral hygiene results than softer bristles?"
    a. "Yes. They do remove more plaque."
    b. "Yes, and they also stimulate the gum tissue."
    c. "No. Actually we used to believe a stiffer brush worked well, but research has given us a wealth of new information. We now believe soft bristles remove much more plaque."
    d. "Actually, the stiffness of the bristle has little to do with plaque removal."

14. Mrs. Cronin's son-in-law, Peter, has returned for a supportive care visit. He has a history of periodontal surgery and has healthy gingiva, large interproximal spaces, and slight plaque deposits. He says he enjoys using a wooden toothpick to clean between his teeth. How should you proceed?
    a. Coach Peter on the effective use of a toothpick.
    b. Substitute a proximal brush for the toothpick.
    c. Demonstrate the benefit of dental tape for the wide embrasure spaces.
    d. Review his toothbrushing technique.

WHERE do I go for more information or support?

evolve

For suggested web sites and agencies, additional readings and resources, and more chapter-specific information, please consult your Evolve Student Resources. Because of the ever-changing nature of the Internet, please keep in mind that web sites listed and their content may change.

CD-ROM

Reference files: As you work through the CD-ROM exercises, you should be able to print reference files and add them to your class materials. *24-5: Interproximal cleaning*, can be saved to your reference files.

HOW can I keep track of my progress toward competence?

As an ongoing picture of progress, record and monitor clinical experiences relating to Chapter 24 content in your Portfolio.

Self-Reflection

On a regular basis, review these experiences (with a faculty member). Identify strengths, weaknesses (not just numbers), and changes that you would incorporate into your clinical care plan now that you have had these experiences.

25 Dental Caries and Caries Management

WHY do I need to know about Dental Caries and Caries Management?

Dental caries continues to be a principal reason for dental treatment and tooth loss. Although the widespread application of topical and systemic fluoride has helped reduce this dental challenge, it has not been able to eliminate the disease completely. One of the primary responsibilities of the dental hygienist is to understand the dental caries process and to educate patients about the cause and treatment and how to manage risk factors that affect this common infectious disease by recommending and using appropriate prevention strategies for each patient visiting the dental practice.

WHAT will I be able to do with this knowledge?

1. Use CAMBRA to assess dental caries risk on a patient.
2. Develop dental caries prevention and disease intervention strategies for a patient, based on CAMBRA.
3. Recommend the appropriate fluoride products for an individual.
4. Select appropriate therapeutic strategies for implementation in the dental office.
5. Establish an appropriate interval for evaluation of the suggested strategies.
6. Work with other oral healthcare providers in the management of dental caries.

HOW do I prepare myself to transfer this knowledge to patient care?

 Go to Chapter 25 content on your CD-ROM or search for "Dental Caries."

CD Exercises

- *25-1: Dental Caries Management by Risk Assessment:* Determine risk factors for the development of dental caries.
- *25-2: Chemical Therapies:* Identify prevention strategies.
- *25-3: Management of a Carious Lesion:* Identify different lesion types and the biggest challenge in treating each.
- *25-4: Management of a Carious Lesion:* Select appropriate therapeutic options for various carious lesions.

Textbook

Review Case Study 25-1, Remineralization of the Early Carious Lesion, and the various case applications throughout the chapter.

For important concepts and application of knowledge, review the tables, figures, and boxed sections in the textbook.

Information that may be especially helpful for clinical transfer and may be used as a clinical resource:

- Box 25-1 provides a good reference for groups of salivary components.
- Box 25-2 and Table 25-2 provide a good reference for lethal and safe doses of fluoride for adults, children, and adolescents.
- Table 25-1 gives a good reference for the approximate composition of enamel and dentin.

HOW do I perform these skills?

evolve

A printable version of this checklist is available on your Evolve Student Resources.
To provide a fluoride application correctly, I will:
- ☐ Select a fluoride tray size.
- ☐ Dispense and place 2 mL of fluoride into trays.
- ☐ Position patient upright in chair.
- ☐ Dry teeth.
- ☐ Insert trays.
- ☐ Insert saliva ejector.
- ☐ Set timer.
- ☐ Observe process.
- ☐ Remove trays.
- ☐ Remove excess fluoride.
- ☐ Instruct patient.

HOW can I more effectively use this knowledge?

Critical Thinking Activities

Use the following worksheet to complete activity #1.
1. Using the fluoride history and clinical examination findings from the CD-ROM patients indicated on

Worksheet #1, identify the sources of fluoride, and review the dental caries history. Compare the two and document your comparisons.

2. Perform the following experiment when you have not consumed food, drink, or gum for 1 hour:
   a. Using a pH narrow-range indicator test strip (pH of 4 to 7), remove a small amount of plaque from your teeth with a toothpick and use it to moisten the strip. Check the pH, and graph your reading.
   b. Eat your favorite sugar-containing candy.
   c. Moisten another pH test strip with your plaque.
   d. Continue this procedure every 10 minutes for 1 hour or until the pH returns to baseline, approximately 7.0.
   e. Repeat the exercise, but this time after eating the candy and checking pH, rinse with water and re-check the pH.

3. Take an egg at room temperature and paint half of it with topical fluoride. Allow the fluoride to dry. Immerse the egg in vinegar overnight (24 hours). Check the results on the egg, and draw conclusions about the effects of fluoride.

Worksheet #1

Record your findings from Critical Thinking Activity #1 in this table. Using the fluoride history and clinical examination data from the CD-ROM patients (listed), evaluate the impact fluoride has had on their dental caries status.

Patient	Fluoride History	Dental Caries History	Current Findings	Observations
Ann Cronin				
William Johnston				
George Burkett				
Elena Guri				
Eva Bjork				
Maria Bjork				
Adolfo Santana				
Subra Mani				

Chapter **25 Dental Caries and Caries Management**

Review Questions

Check your answers against the Answer Key at the back of this Study Guide to assess what you have learned.

1. All the following statements about enamel are true *except* which one?
   a. Enamel is the most mineralized structure in the human body.
   b. Enamel contains carbonated apatite crystals arranged in rods.
   c. Enamel is porous.
   d. Replacement of phosphate ion by carbonate ion increases enamel's strength.

2. When fluorapatite is formed from hydroxyapatite, the fluoride ion substitutes for which one of the following ions?
   a. Hydroxide ion
   b. Phosphate ion
   c. Calcium ion
   d. Magnesium ion
   e. None of the above

3. Fluoride is an antibacterial and anticaries agent. However, ingesting more fluoride than prescribed can cause serious health problems.
   a. Both statements are true.
   b. Both statements are false.
   c. The first statement is true; the second is false.
   d. The second statement is true; the first is false.

4. Salivary analysis for dental caries risk assessment consists of measuring the stimulated salivary flow rate and bacterial loading for both streptococci mutans (SM) and lactobacilli (LB). Placing a restoration in an active lesion does not reduce the bacterial loading in the remainder of the mouth.
   a. Both statements are true.
   b. Both statements are false.
   c. The first statement is true; the second is false.
   d. The first statement is false; the second is true.

5. Which of the following is *not* a mechanism of fluoride action?
   a. Inhibits plaque bacteria
   b. Reduces stains from enamel
   c. Inhibits demineralization
   d. Enhances remineralization and creates fluorapatite-like surface

6. Demineralization is initiated after a rise in pH. Demineralization and remineralization may occur several times a day on the surfaces of teeth.
   a. The first statement is true; the second is false.
   b. The first statement is false; the second is true.
   c. Both statements are true.
   d. Both statements are false.

7. Which of the following components initially protects enamel from the acid of pathogenic bacteria?
   a. Plaque
   b. Pellicle
   c. Interprismatic layer
   d. None of the above

8. Which of the following choices *best* describes the process of demineralization?
   a. Acid-induced dissolution of enamel
   b. Diffusion of ions along their concentration gradients
   c. Active transport of ions into gingival crevicular fluid
   d. Both *a* and *b*
   e. Both *a* and *c*

9. Which of the following factors is the most important in remineralization?
   a. Fluoride
   b. Carbonate
   c. Saliva
   d. Oral hygiene

10. All the following statements about dental caries are true *except* which one?
    a. The cause of dental caries is multifactorial.
    b. Dental caries is a site-specific disease affecting different teeth and different surfaces of teeth.
    c. Dental caries cannot be iatrogenically transferred from one carious site to a previously uninfected site.
    d. The Decayed, Missing, or Filled (DMF) index is the single standard method for assessing dental caries in a population.
    e. Dental caries is an infectious disease that is transmittable from mother to child.

11. In a classic experiment, Keyes and Jordan noted that one strain of hamsters naturally exhibited dental caries, whereas a second strain of hamsters did not. The difference in disease susceptibility occurred when the strains were housed separately but fed the same diet. However, when the investigators housed the strains together in the same cages, both strains exhibited dental caries. What is the most likely explanation for these observations?
    a. Housing the animals together stressed the animals and decreased saliva secretion.
    b. Dental caries pathogens were transmitted from one strain to another.
    c. Alterations in grooming behaviors cause the change in dental caries susceptibility.
    d. Fluoride exposures were decreased in housing the animal strains together.
    e. Eating behaviors changed in the second strain.

WHERE do I go for more information or support?

For suggested web sites and agencies, additional readings and resources, and more chapter-specific information, please consult your Evolve Student Resources. Because of the ever-changing nature of the Internet, please keep in mind that web sites listed and their content may change.

CD-ROM

Reference files: As you work through the CD-ROM exercises, you should be able to print reference files and add them to your class materials. No specific reference files apply to this chapter.

HOW can I keep track of my progress toward competence?

As an ongoing picture of progress, record and monitor clinical experiences relating to Chapter 25 content in your Portfolio.

Self-Reflection

On a regular basis, review these experiences (with a faculty member). Identify strengths, weaknesses (not just numbers), and changes that you would incorporate into your clinical care plan now that you have had these experiences.

26 Dentifrices

WHY do I need to know about Dentifrices?

One of the most frequently asked questions dental hygienists receive from their patients is, "What toothpaste should I be using?" It is imperative that dental hygienists have a clear understanding of the differences between the numerous dentifrices available for consumers and be able to make recommendations based on the needs of the individual patient.

WHAT will I be able to do with this knowledge?

1. Describe the difference between basic and active ingredients in a dentifrice.
2. List active and basic ingredients in dentifrices, and describe their functions.
3. Discuss compatibility of ingredients in a dentifrice and understand the reasons each is critical to the formulation.
4. Describe adverse effects that can be associated with the use of a dentifrice.
5. Explain the process necessary for a new product to receive U.S. Food and Drug Administration approval for marketing.
6. Discuss the process necessary for a product to receive the American Dental Association's Seal of Acceptance.
7. Differentiate between the roles of the U.S. Food and Drug Administration and the American Dental Association in product marketing.
8. Describe the differences between cosmetic approval and therapeutic approval.
9. Describe the different types of studies used to evaluate agents in dentifrices.
10. Explain the process by which a systematic review is conducted.
11. List the agents used in a dentifrice for the treatment of dental caries, sensitivity, gingivitis, calculus, stain removal, whitening, plaque removal, oral malodor, and inflammation.
12. Discuss the history of the evolution of dentifrices.
13. Distinguish between stain removal and whitening.
14. Recommend the appropriate dentifrice for each member of the family in Case Study 26-1.
15. Discuss the ingredients and function of each used in natural dentifrices.

HOW do I prepare myself to transfer this knowledge to patient care?

 Go to Chapter 26 content on your CD-ROM or search for "Dentifrice."

CD Exercises

- *26-1: Composition of a Dentifrice:* Match ingredients to proportions, and save your answers in your reference files.
- *26-2: Composition of a Dentifrice:* Match dentifrice ingredients to function, and save your answers in your reference files.
- *26-3: Dentifrice Formulations—Ann Cronin, George Burkett, William Johnston, Adolfo Santana:* Select a recommended dentifrice based on patient need.

Textbook

Review Case Study 26-1, Selecting an Appropriate Dentifrice, and the case applications.

For important concepts and application of knowledge, review tables, figures, and boxed sections in the textbook.

The following may be especially helpful for clinical transfer and may be used as a clinical resource.

- Table 26-1: Basic Dentifrice Ingredients
- Figure 26-1: Dentifrice Ingredients
- Figure 26-3: Comparison of toothpaste abrasiveness based on relative dentin abrasitivity (RDA)

HOW can I more effectively use this knowledge?

Critical Thinking Activities

Use the following worksheet to complete activities #1 and #2.

1. Using Worksheet #1, survey 20 consumers (i.e., non-dental professionals) to gain insights on purchasing practices of dental products.
2. Using Worksheet #2, go to a local supermarket where you do your grocery shopping. If your dental hygienist sent you to this store and told you to purchase the following products, how many choices would you have in each category? What are the price ranges for each category? What selections would you make, and why?

Worksheet #1

Complete the following worksheet to survey 20 customers.

Name _____

Age _____ □ Male   □ Female

1. Do you recall the last oral care product purchased?
   - □ Yes. If yes, what was it? _____
   - □ No

2. Regarding the last purchase of a dentifrice, do you recall a specific brand name purchased?
   - □ Yes. If yes, what was it? _____
   - □ No

3. Do you recall the type of store where the purchase was made?
   - □ Yes.   □ If yes, what was it?   □ Grocery

     □ Pharmacy

     □ Superstore (e.g., Kmart, Sam's Club, Wal-Mart, etc.)
   - □ No

4. What was your main reason for purchasing that particular brand?
   - □ Professional recommendation
   - □ Price
   - □ Personal preference
   - □ Advice of a friend

5. Do you consider yourself loyal to a specific brand of dentifrice; that is, do you repeatedly purchase the same dentifrice?
   - □ Yes   If yes, what brand? _____
   - □ No

6. If a dental hygienist recommended a specific self-care product to purchase, how likely would you comply?
   - □ Very likely
   - □ Possibly
   - □ Not likely

138

Worksheet #2

Use this worksheet to complete Critical Thinking Activity #2.

Go to a local supermarket where you do your grocery shopping. If your dental hygienist sent you to this store and told you to purchase the following products, how many choices would you have in each category? What are the price ranges for each category? What selections would you make, and why?

Dentifrice Category	Number of Choices	Price Range in Category	Identify Which Product You Would Choose	State Your Reason for Making This Decision
Tartar Control				
Desensitizing				
Whitening				
Remineralizing				
Malodor				
Smoker's Dentifrice				
All Natural Dentifrice				

Continued

Chapter **26** **Dentifrices**

SUMMARY QUESTIONS

Looking at only *one* category, whitening dentifrice, from how many different categories of product would a patient need to choose?

_____

_____

Assuming that a dental professional is not guiding the patient's selection, what factors do you think the patient will use in his or her selection process?

_____

_____

In which dentifrice category did you find the greatest price range?

_____

_____

What factor would you speculate causes this greater price range?

_____

_____

Should price be a consideration in your oral care recommendation?

_____

_____

If yes, why?

_____

_____

If no, why?

_____

_____

What other factors will influence an oral care product selection in the grocery store environment?

_____

_____

DO I have all the answers?

Review Questions

Check your answers against the Answer Key at the back of this Study Guide to assess what you have learned.

1. Currently the ADA Seal of Acceptance is *not* given to any product as being effective against which of the following?
   a. Gingivitis
   b. Periodontitis
   c. Dental caries
   d. Dentin sensitivity
2. A commercial dentifrice can be found in all of the following forms *except* which one?
   a. Paste
   b. Gel
   c. Rinse
   d. Powder
3. People reporting allergic reactions to components of dentifrices are generally reacting to which of the following groups?
   a. Abrasives
   b. Humectants
   c. Flavorings
   d. Coloring agents
4. The ADA Seal of Acceptance is currently administered by which of the following groups?
   a. Council on Dental Research
   b. Council on Scientific Research
   c. Council on Scientific Affairs
   d. Committee of Studies Applications
5. The U.S. Food and Drug Administration regulates marketing of dentifrices by demanding evidence of all of the following *except* which one?
   a. No carcinogenicity
   b. No allergenicity
   c. High customer approval ratings
   d. Proof of effectiveness
6. Large dentifrice trials that compare one active ingredient against another in coded containers are referred to as which one of the following groups?
   a. Efficacy studies
   b. Superiority studies
   c. Placebo-based studies
   d. Pilot studies
7. Stannous fluoride is an effective chemotherapeutic agent for all of the following conditions *except* which one?
   a. Dental caries
   b. Dentin sensitivity
   c. Diminished salivary flow
   d. Gingivitis
8. The anticalculus ingredient that appears to be most effective in dentifrice preparations is which of the following?
   a. Zinc citrate
   b. Sodium hexametaphosphate
   c. Enzymes
   d. Gantrez copolymer

9. Salts used in dentin sensitivity preparations include all of the following *except* which one?
   a. Potassium nitrate
   b. Sodium chloride
   c. Sodium monofluorophosphate
   d. Sodium bicarbonate
10. Nonperoxide-type tooth whiteners act by which of the following mechanisms?
    a. Mild abrasives and polishers along with a tartar-control ingredient
    b. Mildly acidic base material
    c. Enamel-penetrating chemicals
    d. Increased amounts of detergents
11. The most common active ingredient in commercial sensitivity control dentifrices is which of the following?
    a. Sodium monofluorophosphate
    b. Strontium chloride
    c. Sodium citrate
    d. Sodium chloride
    e. Potassium nitrate
12. True whitening dentifrices produce their effect by which of the following?
    a. Abrading the outermost layer of enamel
    b. Dissolving stain
    c. Adding a white coating to the tooth surface
    d. Altering tooth color
13. A dentifrice that has a low relative dentin abrasitivity index number is which of the following?
    a. Low in abrasion
    b. High in abrasion
14. Sodium bicarbonate is effective in reducing oral malodor because it:
    a. Is bactericidal
    b. Inhibits volatile sulfuric compounds
    c. Has a low pH
    d. Is mildly abrasive
15. Xylitol is which of the following?
    a. Naturally occurring
    b. Synthetic

WHERE do I go for more information or support?

evolve

For suggested web sites and agencies, additional readings and resources, and more chapter-specific information, please consult your Evolve Student Resources. Because of the ever-changing nature of the Internet, please keep in mind that web sites listed and their content may change.

 CD-ROM

Reference files: Some of the exercises for Chapter 26 should be written to a reference file once you have completed them:
- 26-1: Composition of a Dentifrice
- 26-2: Composition of a Dentifrice

HOW can I keep track of my progress toward competence?

As an ongoing picture of progress, record and monitor clinical experiences relating to Chapter 26 content in your Portfolio.

Self-Reflection

On a regular basis, review these experiences (with a faculty member). Identify strengths, weaknesses (not just numbers), and changes that you would incorporate into your clinical care plan now that you have had these experiences.

27 Chemotherapeutics

WHY do I need to know about Chemotherapeutics?

The dental hygienist is vital to assessing, diagnosing, and treating periodontal diseases. Many treatment options are available for controlling supragingival and subgingival plaque biofilm. The dental hygienist must stay current regarding evidence-based treatments for gingivitis and periodontitis so that appropriate decisions can be made for individual patients.

WHAT will I be able to do with this knowledge?

1. Discuss the rationale for chemotherapeutic treatments for reducing and controlling plaque biofilm, gingivitis, and other periodontal disease and maintaining periodontal health.
2. Differentiate among chemotherapeutic agents and delivery systems to select the optimal intervention and sequence for patient care.
3. Discuss the evidence base for selecting the various chemotherapeutic agents.
4. Discuss the available chemotherapies and the advantages and disadvantages of each.
5. Discuss the American Dental Association and the U.S. Food and Drug Administration guidelines for accepting chemotherapeutic agents for the control of plaque biofilm, gingivitis, and periodontitis.
6. Discuss the need for and methods of staying informed regarding developments and changes in the standards for using chemotherapeutic agents as adjuncts to nonsurgical periodontal therapy.

HOW do I prepare myself to transfer this knowledge to patient care?

 Go to Chapter 27 content on your CD-ROM or search for "Chemotherapeutics."

CD Exercises

- *27-1: Evaluation of Chemotherapeutic Agents:* Match the agents to the correct mechanism of action, benefits, and side effects.
- *27-2: Control of Plaque Biofilm and Gingivitis with Chemotherapeutic Agents—Ann Cronin, George Burkett, William Johnston, Adolfo Santana:* Answer the case-based questions on several patients for

whom you will make chemotherapeutic recommendations based on specific patient needs, using the oral risk assessment form.

Textbook

Review Case Study 27-1, Selecting a Chemotherapeutic Agent Based on Patient Need, and the case applications. Some considerations to guide your thoughts may include the following:

- Is the level of plaque biofilm control adequate?
- What type of therapy would you recommend?
- Which chemotherapeutic agent would you recommend for the treatment of tooth #10?
- If scaling and root planing of tooth #10 does not improve the probing depth, what options will you suggest for that site?

For important concepts and application of knowledge, review tables, figures, and boxed sections in the textbook.

Boxes and tables in this chapter may be especially helpful for clinical transfer and may be used as clinical resource.

- Box 27-1: Guidelines for Chemotherapeutic Products for Control of Gingivitis
- Box 27-2: Guidelines for Chemotherapeutic Agents to Slow or Arrest Periodontitis
- Box 27-3: Tips for Arestin Tip Placement
- Box 27-4: Potential Concerns with Systemic Antimicrobials
- Box 27-5: Most Commonly Prescribed Antibiotics in Dentistry
- Table 27-1: Comparison of Topically Applied Antigingivitis Agents
- Table 27-2: Mouthrinses: Adverse Effects, Precautions, and Contraindications
- Table 27-3: U.S. Food and Drug Administration Pregnancy Classifications

HOW can I more effectively use this knowledge?

Critical Thinking Activities

Use the following worksheets to complete your activity #3.

1. Go to the American Dental Association (ADA) web site (www.ada.org), and study the list of products that have the ADA Seal of Acceptance.

143

2. Watch instructional videotapes on manipulating various chemotherapeutic delivery systems. Using a typodont, practice the insertion techniques with gels, irrigation, chips, and powders.

3. Obtain the drug insert sheet on different oral antimicrobial agents. These items are frequently available on the Internet. Compare the recommendations for use, advantages and disadvantages, and reported precautions. Record your findings on Worksheet #1 and Worksheet #2.

4. Develop a brochure for the patient to take home on each of the controlled drug-delivery systems. Such information may be obtained directly from the manufacturer, the company's web site, or the package insert.

5. Track the efficacy of each intervention used in Critical Thinking Activity #4.

6. With the aid of a microbiologist, culture saliva or plaque biofilm. Investigate the effects of various antimicrobials. (Saliva is easier to culture than plaque biofilm.)

7. Role-play with a student partner the roles of Ms. Tevus (from Case Study 27-1) and the dental hygienist. Explain the role a chemotherapeutic agent might play in Ms. Tevus's oral health.

8. Use the American Academy of Periodontology (AAP) web site (www.perio.org) to access position papers pertaining to the use of pharmacotherapeutics in treating periodontal diseases.

9. Select one chemotherapeutic agent to research in-depth and report to your class.

Worksheet #1

Use Worksheets #1 and #2 to record your responses to Critical Thinking Activity #3.

Oral Antimicrobial Agent	Also Known As (AKA) (Product Name)	Recommended Use	Advantages	Disadvantages	Reported Precautions
Minocycline microspheres					
Chlorhexidine gluconate	Perio Chip				
Tetracycline					
Doxycycline hyclate					

Chapter **27 Chemotherapeutics**

Worksheet #2

Complete the table below with the adverse effects, precautions, and contraindications of the listed chemotherapeutic agents.

Agent	Adverse Effects	Precautions	Contraindications
Water			
Chlorhexidine digluconate (CHX)			
Essential oils			
SnF^2			
Triclosan			
Sanguinarine			
Oxygenating agents			
Baking soda, salt, and hydrogen peroxide			
Quaternary ammonium compounds			
Povidone-iodine			
Prebrushing rinses			

DO I have all the answers?

Review Questions

Check your answers against the Answer Key at the back of this Study Guide to assess what you have learned.

The following review questions refer to Case Study 27-1.

1. For the profile that does not indicate an increase in generalized bleeding, which one of the following approaches would you select for Ms. Tevus at this appointment?
   a. Schedule her for care every 2 months instead of at 3-month intervals.
   b. Take a sample to culture for suspected periodontal pathogens.
   c. Place her on a pulsed-water irrigator.
   d. Refer her to the periodontist.

2. Which one of the following types of infection do you suspect that Ms. Tevus has?
   a. Necrotizing ulcerative gingivitis
   b. Plaque biofilm–associated periodontitis
   c. Linear gingival erythema
   d. Hormonal gingivitis

3. Which one of the following conditions seems to be Ms. Tevus's most obvious problem?
   a. Inadequate plaque biofilm control
   b. Noncompliance
   c. An immunocompromised system
   d. Stress

4. What adjunctive therapy would you recommend for Ms. Tevus to assist in controlling plaque biofilm and gingivitis?
   a. Locally administered antibiotic or antimicrobial (LAA) therapy
   b. Approved antigingivitis daily mouthrinse
   c. Floss holder
   d. Brushing with a fluoridated toothpaste

5. Which mouthrinse would you recommend for adjunctive treatment of plaque biofilm and gingivitis?
   a. Essential oil
   b. Chlorhexidine digluconate (CHX)
   c. Stannous fluoride
   d. Prebrushing rinse
   e. Either *a* or *b*

6. What other options are available for Ms. Tevus to control plaque biofilm and gingivitis?
   a. Irrigate with stannous fluoride
   b. Add a toothpaste with triclosan
   c. Use LAA therapy
   d. Recommend stress therapy

7. Which one of the following treatment options would you consider for tooth #10?
   1. Provide debridement only.
   2. Wait and see what changes irrigation might produce.

3. Use local delivery therapy such as minocycline microspheres, CHX chip, or doxycycline hyclate.
   4. Refer the patient to a periodontist.
   a. All of the above
   b. *3* only
   c. *2, 3,* and *4*
   d. *4* only

8. If LAAs were used on tooth #10 and the site did not resolve after the first attempt, what would be the next treatment option?
   1. Provide debridement.
   2. Place the LAA in the site.
   3. Instruct the patient about the need for immaculate home care.
   4. Refer the patient to a periodontist.
   a. *1, 2,* and *3*
   b. *4* only
   c. All of the above
   d. *2* only

WHERE do I go for more information or support?

evolve

For suggested web sites and agencies, additional readings and resources, and more chapter-specific information, please consult your Evolve Student Resources. Because of the ever-changing nature of the Internet, please keep in mind that web sites listed and their content may change.

CD-ROM

Reference files: As you work through the CD-ROM exercises, you should be able to print reference files and add them to your class materials. No specific reference files apply to this chapter.

HOW can I keep track of my progress toward competence?

As an ongoing picture of progress, record and monitor clinical experiences relating to Chapter 27 content in your Portfolio.

Self-Reflection

On a regular basis, review these experiences (with a faculty member). Identify strengths, weaknesses (not just numbers), and changes that you would incorporate into your clinical care plan now that you have had these experiences.

28 Sealants

WHY do I need to know about Sealants?

Dental caries is considered an infectious, transmissible disease. The Centers for Disease Control and Prevention report that dental caries is possibly the most prevalent infectious disease in American children. Dental caries is five times more common than asthma and seven times more common than hay fever in children (U.S. Department of Health and Human Services: *Oral Health in America: A Report of the Surgeon General,* Rockville, Md., 2000, U.S. Department of Health and Human Services, National Institute of Dental and Craniofacial Research, National Institutes of Health). The need to assess and recognize dental caries at its earliest stage is critical in preventing future restorative treatment. The dental hygienist is a specialist in preventing oral diseases and is in a primary role to assess a patient's risk for dental caries. The dental hygienist can recommend specific strategies, including the placement of dental sealants, to promote dental health.

WHAT will I be able to do with this knowledge?

1. Recognize that sealants are a primary preventive means of reducing the need for future restorative treatment.
2. Discuss the types and general properties of dental sealant materials, including potential estrogenicity.
3. Discuss the indications for using pit and fissure sealants.
4. List the criteria for selecting teeth for the placement of sealant materials.
5. Using and applying the dental caries risk assessment principles, assess a patient's dental caries risk, and determine the need for sealant placement.
6. Describe how sealant materials are retained in the pits and fissures of enamel surfaces.
7. Describe the appropriate application technique of sealant materials.
8. Describe the efficacy and cost-effectiveness of dental sealants.
9. Apply the principles of sealant placement to clinical dental hygiene experiences.
10. Cite three reasons for dental practitioners' underuse of sealants.

HOW do I prepare myself to transfer this knowledge to patient care?

 Go to Chapter 28 content on your CD-ROM or search for "Dental Sealants."

CD Exercises

- *28-1: Indication for Dental Sealant Placement—Terrence Zellar:* Make sealant recommendations based on patient needs and records for Terrence Zellar.
- *28-2: Armamentarium and Application:* Complete the order of steps in sealant placement for review.
- *28-3: Armamentarium and Application:* Select the correct armamentarium for a sealant procedure.
- *28-4: Armamentarium and Application—Subra Mani:* Make sealant recommendations based on patient needs and records for Subra Mani.

Textbook

Review the Case Study 28-1, Pediatric Considerations for Sealant Application, and the case applications. After reading the chapter, consider the following:
- Complete a dental caries risk assessment on Meghan Kopel and be sure to include an analysis of the patient's dietary patterns and current and past fluoride exposure.

For important concepts and application of knowledge, review tables, figures, and boxed sections in the textbook.

Elements in this chapter that may be especially helpful for clinical transfer and may be used as clinical resources:
- Box 28-1: Factors in Sealant Placement
- Box 28-3: Armamentarium for Sealant Application
- Box 28-4: Application Technique for Dental Sealant

HOW do I perform these skills?

evolve

A printable version of this checklist is available on your Evolve Student Resources.
To ensure proper sealant application, I will:
- ☐ Obtain proper armamentarium.
- ☐ Cleanse the tooth surfaces of hard and soft debris with a prophylaxis brush on a slow-speed hand piece or with an air polisher.

□ Thoroughly rinse conditioning agent.

□ Properly isolate the tooth to prevent any moisture contamination.

□ Apply the phosphoric acid enamel conditioner covering all areas of the enamel surface to be sealed.

□ Thoroughly rinse cleansing agent.

□ Thoroughly dry tooth surface.

□ Evaluate the tooth surfaces for a frosty-white appearance over the areas to be sealed.

□ Apply the sealant material according to the manufacturer's directions.

□ Polymerize the sealant through either light or chemical curing.

□ Examine the sealant for voids, undercuring, and proper extension into pits and fissures.

□ Evaluate the patient's occlusion with the use of articulating paper.

□ Smooth any high areas with a slow-speed hand piece and finishing bur or fine stone.

□ Before patient dismissal administer a neutral sodium fluoride treatment to ensure remineralization of the previously etched tooth surfaces.

□ Set patient or parent expectations (outcomes).

□ Document findings and procedures in chart.

HOW can I more effectively use this knowledge?

Critical Thinking Activities

Use the following worksheet to complete activity #4.

1. Practice sealant placement on a typodont, extracted teeth, or a peer.
2. Organize or participate in a dental health fair. Develop pamphlets on dental pit and fissure sealants and dental caries prevention.
3. Develop a table clinic on the use of dental sealants in the prevention of decay.
4. Organize and promote sealant and education programs for an elementary school. Record all information on Worksheet #1.
5. Compare and contrast the retention of dental sealants with various methods of enamel preparation on extracted teeth: pumice only, acid-etch technique, air abrasion, fluoride application before sealant placement, and enameloplasty.

Worksheet #1

Use this worksheet with Critical Thinking Activity #4.

An elementary school has asked your dental hygiene class to organize a sealant program for second graders. Using the form and information here, develop a community-based dental sealant program.

Your class can provide five dental hygiene students and one faculty member in 4-hour rotations of time, once per week, to administer the program.

Name of school: Greenwood Elementary

Number of students: 238

Number of classes involved: 10

Number (approximate) of first molars to be sealed: _____

Amount of time required per child to place sealants: _____

Total time required to administer program: _____

Number of dental hygiene students needed: _____

Amount of sealant material needed: _____

All armamentarium required:

Item	Total Quantity
_____	_____
_____	_____
_____	_____
_____	_____
_____	_____
_____	_____
_____	_____

Written materials to be developed (remember permission slips, parental education, information and education for teachers and children, and a press release):

_____

_____

DO I have all the answers?

Review Questions

Check your answers against the Answer Key at the back of this Study Guide to assess what you have learned. Question 4 refers to Case Study 28-1.

1. Proper acid-etch bonding produces which of the following bonds?
   a. Mechanical
   b. Chemical
   c. Both *a* and *b*
   d. None of the above
2. Which of the following best explains the underuse of sealants?
   a. Retention rate of sealants
   b. Fear of dental caries being buried under sealant
   c. Cost-effectiveness of the procedure
   d. All of the above
3. A 20-year-old female patient comes to your office for prophylaxis. She is primarily interested in having her teeth polished and requests that you use an air-powder polisher. She has sealants on all her molars and premolars. Which of the following statements is correct regarding air-polishing of sealants?
   a. It does not harm pit and fissure sealants provided the power is on a low setting.
   b. It does not result in changes to the sealant surface.
   c. It is safe to use as a cleansing method before sealant placement.
   d. It is not contraindicated for use on resin sealants.
4. Approximately 3 months after Meghan's sealants were placed, none of the sealants were clinically evident (see Case Study 28-1). What is the most likely cause for the early loss of these materials?
   a. The etched enamel site was contaminated by oil or water in the compressed air used for drying.
   b. Light wand was held too closely to the sealant surface.
   c. Sealant was overexposed to light polymerization.
   d. The acid etchant used was at a concentration of 40%.
5. At recall examinations, sealants may have a brown stain along some marginal areas. Which of the following is the cause of this finding?
   a. Inadequate enamel preparation at margin
   b. Contamination of site
   c. Overextension of sealant beyond etched preparation
   d. Occlusal forces producing stress at thin areas of sealant, exceeding bond strength
   e. All of the above

6. One year after sealant placement, the dental hygienist's clinical examination reveals that the sealants on teeth #3 and #14 are only partially intact. Both teeth are missing resin from the palatal groove. Which of the following statements is correct to replace the missing areas?
   a. After scaling, cleanse the area, etch, dry, and apply the resin material.
   b. After scaling and polishing, etch, dry, and place the resin sealant.
   c. Air-polish the entire tooth for 30 seconds, then place the resin sealant.

WHERE do I go for more information or support?

evolve

For suggested web sites and agencies, additional readings and resources, and more chapter-specific information, please consult your Evolve Student Resources. Because of the ever-changing nature of the Internet, please keep in mind that web sites listed and their content may change.

CD-ROM

Reference files: As you work through the CD-ROM exercises, you should be able to print reference files and add them to your class materials. No specific reference files apply to this chapter.

HOW can I keep track of my progress toward competence?

As an ongoing picture of progress, record and monitor clinical experiences relating to Chapter 28 content in your Portfolio.

Self-Reflection

On a regular basis, review these experiences (with a faculty member). Identify strengths, weaknesses (not just numbers), and changes that you would incorporate into your clinical care plan now that you have had these experiences.

29 Tobacco Dependence and Addictive Behaviors

WHY do I need to know about Tobacco Dependence and Addictive Behaviors?

Addictive behaviors and the products that cause them significantly affect the practice of dental hygiene in numerous ways. Learning to connect the risks and associated substance-specific chronic, progressive, and relapsing challenges associated with addictions can help dental hygienists educate and support their patients through the challenges of cessation and improving overall health.

WHAT will I be able to do with this knowledge?

1. Recognize various ways that tobacco use undermines oral health and dental practice.
2. Recognize that nicotine and other chemical dependencies are chronic, progressive, and relapsing conditions of the brain, which alter vital neural functions.
3. Recognize common symptoms of nicotine and other drug dependencies and withdrawal.
4. Recognize that nicotine dependency can be effectively treated with modest, scientifically established methods and periodic reinforcement.
5. Use basic behavioral and pharmacotherapeutic intervention services in clinical practice.
6. Establish clinic policies and practices that ensure routine identification of patient tobacco use status and appropriate methods for care and follow-up.
7. Refer selected patients for specialized treatment of their nicotine and other drug dependencies.

HOW do I prepare myself to transfer this knowledge to patient care?

 Go to Chapter 29 content on your CD-ROM or search for "Tobacco Cessation."

CD Exercises

- *29-1: Techniques, Procedures and Support Treatment— Subra Mani:* Determine an appropriate tobacco cessation program for patient.

Textbook

Review Case Study 29-1, Helping a Patient Quit Tobacco Use.

In situations in which multiple case applications that will bring this case study to life also exist, use this information to think of ways you might discuss these important issues with your patients in clinic.

For important concepts and application of knowledge, review tables, figures, and boxed sections in the book.

The following boxes may be especially helpful for clinical transfer and may be used as clinical resources:

- Box 29-1: Tobacco-Induced and Tobacco-Associated Oral Conditions. This reference is good for reminding you of oral conditions to be aware of in your patients who use tobacco or other addictive elements.
- Box 29-2: Tobacco Effects on Clinical Care. This reference is good for reminding you of the effects tobacco may have on the care you will provide, as well as the variations in outcome that you can anticipate with patients who smoke.
- Box 29-4: American Psychiatric Association: Diagnostic Criteria for Nicotine Withdrawal. This reference is good for remembering personally, as well as for supporting your patients who are trying to quit and experience these symptoms.
- Box 29-5: U.S. Food and Drug Administration: Approved Tobacco-Cessation Pharmaceutical Agents. This reference is excellent as you make recommendations and discuss the issues of tobacco cessation with patients.

HOW do I perform these skills?

evolve

A printable version of this checklist is available on your Evolve Student Resources.
To identify tobacco use and respond appropriately, I will be able to:

- ☐ Ask the patient whether he or she uses any form of tobacco.
- ☐ Advise the patient to stop.
- ☐ Assist the patient in successful quitting.
    - ☐ Have the patient set a quit date.
    - ☐ Encourage the patient to deal with one stressor at a time.
- ☐ Arrange follow-up contacts.
- ☐ Help the patient:
    - ☐ Cope with physical withdrawal, including possible depression
    - ☐ Cope with environmental cues to smoke

□ Cope with deeply ingrained habits
□ Cope with other common relapse risks
□ Provide the patient with two items:
□ A slip of paper to remind the patient at home of the quit date the patient chooses
□ A booklet that will help the patient prepare for their quit date
□ Document findings and procedure in chart.

HOW can I more effectively use this knowledge?

Critical Thinking Activities

Use the following worksheets to complete activities #3 and #4.

1. Develop a presentation for elementary school students about the brain functions that occur to develop a chemical dependency.
2. Review a group of 10 clinic patient records at random. Identify the number using tobacco and the type of product. Look for any notation as to whether quitting was discussed with the patient and what the outcome or decision was at that time. Keep notes of this activity.
3. Go to a grocery store, convenience mart, and another type of store that sells tobacco products. Identify where tobacco products are kept and whether signage about age restrictions on purchasing tobacco products is displayed. On Worksheet #1, record the amount of time you spend in the store, the number of tobacco products customers purchased while you were there, and the approximate age of the purchaser.
4. Interview three people: someone who has quit smoking more than 3 years ago, someone who has recently quit, and someone who has committed to quitting. Ask questions of each person about concerns about quitting, successes for those who have quit, support needed to quit, and what got them through the desire to continue use. For the person who has committed to quit, ask about expectations of behavior and means of coping during this time. Record your findings on Worksheet #2.
5. Complete the following multipart exercise.
   a. Ask friends who use tobacco why they do it and what their thoughts and intentions are about doing so in the future. Do not be judgmental. Use your listening skills. Develop a list that shows responses under headings by type, for example, as follows:

Liking tobacco

Taste, smell, feel, color of container
Image: helps to appear to be like someone else
Ability to manage mood: relief of stress, thinking
Helps in weight control
Helps in social situations
No reasons for using

Not liking tobacco

Cost
Image
Taste, smell, feel, etc.
Feeling of not being in control
Health concerns
Other reasons

Interest in quitting

Not interested at all
Somewhat interested
Interested a lot
Interested and have tried to quit before

Experience in trying to quit

How long they were abstinent
How the quitting process felts
How many of these individuals used a nicotine replacement product or other pharmacologic aid? Did it make a difference? What caused relapses: physical, social, other?

   b. Ask individuals whether they would like you to help them quit. Keep track of what percentage of those you ask agree to quit with your help.
   c. Help interested friends quit. Help them identify as many reasons as possible for wanting to quit. Talk with them about concerns while quitting, such as experiencing physical withdrawal, stress, weight gain, and other common side effects during the recovery process. Help them identify social situations, places, and conditions that are most likely to tempt them to relapse, and offer suggestions about how they might deal with these temptations. Try the different methods suggested in this chapter and think of others. (The chapter cannot cover all common possibilities or anticipate every situation that people confront.) Of course, if a prescription drug is desired, the tobacco user's physician or dentist would have to be consulted. If possible, try to be supportive and positive over at least the first 3 months after your friend quits.
   d. Encourage friends who relapse to try again.
   e. Check to see how the tobacco-use status of each clinic patient is determined, and learn the system used to encourage users and help them quit.

These experiences help you learn in an informal, systematic way about the ways tobacco influences people and the obstacles they face when they are trying to quit. Few acts of friendship or professionalism can be stronger than helping someone break free from tobacco use. Success, even limited abstinence, reduces their chances of experiencing tobacco-related health problems, including oral health problems, and the possibility of an entirely avoidable premature death.

Worksheet #1

Use the following form to record your findings from Critical Thinking Activity #3.

Location of Products	Grocery Store	Drug Store	Convenience Mart
Age restriction signage			
Types of Products Sold			
Cut			
Chew			
Snuff			
Cigarettes			
Cigars			
Bidis			
Kretek			
Pipe			
Number of tobacco products sold in 30 minutes			
Average age of purchasers (estimate)			
Gender of purchasers			

155

Worksheet #2

Use the following form to record your findings from Critical Thinking Activity #4.

	Quit Smoking More Than 3 Years	Recently Quit Smoking	Committed To Quit
Concerns over quitting			
Success stories or strategies			
Support needed now and future			
What got them through, or what they will need to get them through			
Expectations of behavior			
Means of coping			

DO I have all the answers?

Review Questions

Check your answers against the Answer Key at the back of this Study Guide to assess what you have learned.

1. On which one of the following areas does nicotine act directly?
   a. Sympathetic nervous system
   b. Neuromuscular junction
   c. Medulla of the adrenal cortex
   d. Brain
   e. All of the above

2. Which one of the following characteristics best describes nicotine?
   a. Not addictive
   b. Not as addictive as heroin and cocaine
   c. As addictive as heroin and cocaine
   d. More addictive than heroin and cocaine
   e. Addictive and the most harmful substance in tobacco

3. Tobacco use is a strong risk factor for all *except* which one of the following conditions?
   a. Periodontal diseases
   b. Tooth loss
   c. Oral cancer
   d. Gingival bleeding
   e. Halitosis

4. Which one of the following options best describes the effect of tobacco-using patients on dental practices compared with tobacco-free patients?
   a. Greater loss of patients as users succumb to tobacco-related diseases
   b. Greater number of appointment cancellations
   c. Greater need to consult with patients' physicians
   d. Greater risk of in-treatment emergency care
   e. All of the above

5. Which one of the following options describes the oral health team's role in helping patients quit using tobacco?
   a. It is not as effective as medical teams.
   b. It is about equally effective as medical teams.
   c. It is more effective than medical teams.
   d. It is ineffective.
   e. It is of unknown effectiveness.

6. All *except* which one of the following actions describe routine clinical steps in helping patients quit using tobacco?
   a. Asking patients about tobacco use and experience with quitting
   b. Advising patients, showing them examples of tobacco-related oral conditions and reinforcing their reasons to quit
   c. Attacking patients' misperceptions
   d. Assisting with coping skills and planning strategies
   e. Arranging follow-up in support of the quitting and recovery process

7. Which one of the following combinations of agents has been helpful during the quitting process?
   a. Nicotine gum, nasal spray, suppository, and inhaler
   b. Nicotine gum, patch, nasal spray, and bupropion (Wellbutrin)
   c. Nicotine gum, patch, nasal spray, inhaler, and buspirone
   d. Nicotine gum, patch, inhaler, and bupropion (Wellbutrin)
   e. Smokeless tobacco

8. All of the following actions are predictors of relapse while trying to quit except one. Which one is the *exception?*
   a. A spouse who uses tobacco
   b. Taking a single puff from a cigarette
   c. Moderate alcohol use
   d. Feelings of depression
   e. Having quit before but relapsed

9. Follow-up contacts with the patient should occur just before the quit date and at another time. Which one of the following instances is the other time the clinician should contact the patient?
   a. At least at the end of each of the first 3 months
   b. During the first few days and monthly during pharmacotherapy
   c. On the quit date and at monthly intervals
   d. Whenever the patient requests it
   e. Every 6 months for life

10. The American Dental Association performs all of the following activities to encourage the oral health team to help patients avoid and discontinue tobacco use except one. Which one is the *exception?*
    a. Adopting policies that encourage clinical tobacco-intervention services
    b. Including tobacco counseling in its standard procedure codes
    c. Publishing tobacco company advertising in its journals and newsletters
    d. Describing approved drugs for tobacco cessation in its *Guide to Dental Therapeutics*
    e. Including a tobacco question in the American Dental Association health history form

WHERE do I go for more information or support?

evolve

For suggested web sites and agencies, additional readings and resources, and more chapter-specific information, please consult your Evolve Student Resources. Because of the ever-changing nature of the Internet, please keep in mind that web sites listed and their content may change.

CD-ROM

Reference files: As you work through the CD-ROM exercises, you should be able to print reference files and add them to your class materials. No specific reference files apply to this chapter.

Chapter **29** **Tobacco Dependence and Addictive Behaviors**

HOW can I keep track of my progress toward competence?

As an ongoing picture of progress, record and monitor clinical experiences relating to Chapter 29 content in your Portfolio:

Keep a record of all patients with whom you have discussed tobacco cessation. Review strategies and outcomes to determine methods most effective for you and your patients.

Keep copies of patient information brochures and support materials for quick reference resources for your clinic.

Make a copy of the boxed items in the chapter that can be good resources and reference information for your clinic.

Self-Reflection

On a regular basis, review these experiences (with a faculty member). Identify strengths, weaknesses (not just numbers), and changes that you would incorporate into your clinical care plan now that you have had these experiences.

30 Care of Appliances and Dental Prostheses

WHY do I need to know about the Care of Appliances and Dental Prostheses?

Dental practices vary with respect to the role the dental hygienist is expected to play in educating patients about the care of intraoral appliances. Although the majority of a dental hygienist's training and professional practice is generally devoted to removing deposits from the teeth, patient education in oral health is an important and indispensable duty. The large number of patients with oral prosthetic appliances—dentures, bridges, splints, and orthodontic devices—must be taught and periodically reminded of the techniques for and importance of proper care of their appliances. In addition, the dental hygienist plays an essential role in the assessment of the integrity of such devices and the tissues they contact and in the referral of developing and extant problems before they worsen.

WHAT will I be able to do with this knowledge?

1. Correctly identify the following dental appliances: fixed partial denture, removable partial denture, complete removable denture, overdenture, splint, fluoride tray, bleaching tray, and maxillofacial prosthesis.
2. Practice role-playing a dental hygienist in assessing a patient with fixed and removable prosthetic replacements.
3. Detail the instruments, products, and procedures that are used to clean removable dental prostheses.
4. Explain the need for daily self-care of implant abutments, and specify how and why particular care must be taken.
5. Correctly identify and explain the cause of soft tissue pathoses associated with improperly maintained dental prostheses.
6. Explain to a patient the reason and method for cleaning a dental appliance and the abutment teeth, regardless of whether the appliance is fixed, removable, implant-borne, therapeutic, or prosthetic.

HOW do I prepare myself to transfer this knowledge to patient care?

 Go to Chapter 30 content on your CD-ROM or search for "Dental Appliances."

CD Exercises

- *30-1: Overview of Dental Appliances:* Match appropriate method of care to dental appliance.
- *30-2: Overview of Dental Appliances—Ann Cronin:* Evaluate appliance care, based on patient records.

Textbook

Review the Case Study 30-1, Caring for the Prosthodontic Patient. As you read through the chapter, determine the steps you would take when caring for this patient and the prosthetic devices (that is, the overdenture and the sleep apnea device).

This complex, true-to-life case study highlights the need to evaluate carefully all aspects of patient behavior before making oral self-care recommendations involving prosthodontic appliances.

For important concepts and application of knowledge, review tables, figures, and boxed sections in the textbook.

The following figures may be especially helpful for clinical transfer and may be used as a clinical resource:

- Figures 30-4 through 30-10 show images of various prosthetic appliances.
- Figures 30-11 through 30-15 show intraoral lesions associated with appliances.

HOW do I perform these skills?

evolve

A printable version of this checklist is available on your Evolve Student Resources.

To complete the care of appliances and dental prostheses successfully, I will be able to:

- ☐ Give professional care.
  - ☐ Remove appliance or prosthesis.
  - ☐ Check for loose teeth, chipped saddle areas, broken clasps, and debris.
  - ☐ Show patient technique for debris removal, as appropriate.
  - ☐ Place appliance or prosthesis in a self-closing plastic bag with stain and tartar remover.
  - ☐ Place appliance or prosthesis in ultrasonic and run for appropriate length of time.
  - ☐ Remove appliance or prosthesis from bag.
  - ☐ Remove remaining soft and hard deposits with either a denture brush or dental instrument, as needed.
  - ☐ Rinse appliance thoroughly with water.

159

- □ Rinse appliance with a mouthrinse to freshen it.
- □ Deliver appliance or prosthesis to patient at completion of treatment.
- □ Review patient oral-care instructions.
- □ Set patient expectations (outcomes).
- □ Document findings and procedure in chart.
  - □ Give patient oral care instructions.
    - □ Remove prosthesis after every meal to rinse off adherent food.
    - □ Remove prosthesis each night.
    - □ Clean prosthesis under running water with appropriate denture brush.
    - □ Clean prosthesis over a sink filled with several inches of water or washcloth (to prevent damage if dropped).
    - □ Soak or clean prosthesis with a foaming denture cleansing paste or soaking agent, if needed.

HOW can I more effectively use this knowledge?

Critical Thinking Activities

Use the following worksheet to complete your activity #1.

1. Visit a dental laboratory. Examine dentures as they are repaired and relined. What clues suggest whether the patient was effective at keeping the prosthesis clean? What methods do you suggest to clean the prosthesis before it is returned to the patient? What methods would you suggest to the patient to keep the prosthesis clean in the future? Record your findings on Worksheet #1.

2. At a dentist's office, examine the different designs of the pontics and the connectors of fixed partial dentures that have not yet been delivered to patients. Can you identify designs that would be easier than others for a patient to keep clean? For each case, what would be the device or material you would suggest to the patient to use at home to keep the new prosthesis clean?

3. Obtain some scrap orthodontic wire. Place it in a glass cup with a solution of 9 oz of water and 1 oz of laundry bleach so that some of the wire is covered by liquid and some is not. Keep the wire in the solution for a week. How does the wire look at the end of the week?

4. Obtain a sample of denture cleanser (or buy a small package). Place a tablet of the material in a clear glass of water. What changes does the solution undergo during the next 20 minutes? How does this example differ from what happens to a sample of a different denture cleanser?

5. Repeat Critical Thinking Activity #4, but moisten a polished piece of dental acrylic with water. How does the wetted acrylic feel to your fingers? Now, drop the acrylic into one of the cleansing solutions for several minutes. Remove the acrylic with your fingers. How does it feel now? How long do you need to rinse the acrylic in tap water before the solution's odor disappears? How long is it before the surface of the acrylic feels as it did before it was placed in the cleaning solution? How will this information help you educate patients?

6. Demonstrate the use of tufted floss, such as superfloss, and a proxabrush to a patient who has just received a fixed bridge. When you next see that patient, compare the tendency for gingival bleeding around the prosthesis with the soft tissue behavior of another patient with a bridge who has not been instructed in using these products.

7. The next time you treat a patient who has a removable prosthesis, carefully examine both the tissue surface of the denture and the color and consistency of the mucosa on which it rested. What connection can you make between the appearances of the two?

Worksheet #1

Use the following form with Critical Thinking Activity #1. For each of the procedures listed on this form, record your observations. Try to observe as many aspects of each procedure as possible. State the aspect of the procedure you observed and record your observations. Determine also what infection control measures are or should be in place.

Crown Fabrication

All gold (metal) _____

All porcelain _____

Porcelain fused to gold (metal) _____

Infection control necessary _____

Bridge Fabrication

All gold (metal) _____

All porcelain _____

Porcelain fused to gold (metal) _____

Infection control necessary _____

Veneer Fabrication

Infection control necessary _____

Removable Partial Denture

New _____

Repair _____

Infection control necessary _____

Full Denture

New _____

Repair _____

Infection control necessary _____

Mouth Guard

Infection control necessary _____

Occlusal Guard

Infection control necessary _____

Retainer

Infection control necessary _____

Other

_____

Chapter **30** **Care of Appliances and Dental Prostheses**

DO I have all the answers?

Review Questions

Check your answers against the Answer Key at the back of this Study Guide to assess what you have learned. The following questions refer to Case Study 30-1.

1. Which one of the following options is the most likely reason that the metal framework of Dr. Basha's mandibular removal partial denture (RPD) is dark and dull?
   a. Dr. Basha fails to clean the RPD on a regular basis.
   b. One of the medications Dr. Basha uses probably causes the staining.
   c. The metal framework is an alloy of inferior quality.
   d. Dr. Basha soaks the partial denture too long in a commercial denture-cleansing solution.

2. Which one of the following options is the most likely reason that Dr. Basha dislikes the flavor of the fluoride solution?
   a. It is a neutral sodium-fluoride preparation.
   b. It is a stannous fluoride preparation.
   c. The solution is outdated.
   d. Dr. Basha may not clean the fluoride carrier between uses.

3. For which one of the following arches has the fluoride carrier been prepared?
   a. The maxillary arch, to limit the effect of plaque biofilm on the implant abutments
   b. The mandibular arch, to prevent and remineralize incipient dental caries and to inhibit periodontal pathogens
   c. Either arch, because the increased concentration of fluoride in the oral cavity is effective throughout the mouth
   d. The maxillary arch, to limit the effect of the overdenture on the palatal tissues

4. The tissue underneath the implant splint bar is inflamed for which one of the following reasons?
   a. Tissues beneath dentures are generally inflamed because of the pressure of the prosthesis.
   b. The presence of plaque biofilm between the splint bar and the mucosa is irritating to the soft tissue.
   c. Dr. Basha is likely allergic to nickel in the alloy of the splint bar.
   d. The tight fit of the overdenture causes blood to be brought to the surface of the mucosa whenever the appliance is removed.

5. Which one of the following oral findings in a prosthodontic patient would you associate with Dr. Basha's dry mouth?
   a. The dentures are likely to be clean because so little saliva is present.
   b. The soft tissues beneath the dentures are likely to be inflamed because underhydrated acrylic is toxic.

   c. The soft tissues beneath the dentures are likely to be white and hyperkeratotic because underlubricated prostheses are more retentive.
   d. The soft tissues beneath the dentures are likely to display changes that are consistent with candidal infection because of the absence of saliva and its antimicrobial and lubricant properties.

6. Dr. Basha displays evidence of prior periodontal surgery. For which one of the following reasons would you not insist on him using dental floss on the lower teeth?
   a. He does an acceptable job with an interproximal cleaner.
   b. Dental floss may not be the best device for cleaning beneath a fixed bridge, depending on the contour of the undersurfaces of the contact area and pontics.
   c. Dr. Basha's medical condition dictates the use of a nonfloss alternative.
   d. All of the above.

WHERE do I go for more information or support?

evolve

For suggested web sites and agencies, additional readings and resources, and more chapter-specific information, please consult your Evolve Student Resources. Because of the ever-changing nature of the Internet, please keep in mind that web sites listed and their content may change.

 CD-ROM

Reference files: As you work through the CD-ROM exercises, you should be able to print reference files and add them to your class materials. No specific reference files apply to this chapter.

HOW can I keep track of my progress toward competence?

As an ongoing picture of progress, record and monitor clinical experiences relating to Chapter 30 content in your Portfolio.

Self-Reflection

On a regular basis, review these experiences (with a faculty member). Identify strengths, weaknesses (not just numbers), and changes that you would incorporate into your clinical care plan now that you have had these experiences.

31 Powered Instrumentation and Periodontal Debridement

WHY do I need to know about Powered Instrumentation and Periodontal Debridement?

Periodontal debridement is the foundation of treatment offered by the dental hygienist. The goals of periodontal debridement are to arrest infection and maintain a healthy periodontium by eliminating the pathogenic microorganisms on the tooth and root surface and removing hardened calculus deposits and dental plaque biofilm from the sulcus or pocket.

WHAT will I be able to do with this knowledge?

1. Make appropriate instrument selections—manual or powered—for periodontal debridement.
2. Discuss the process of pathogenesis and wound healing relative to the need for periodontal debridement.
3. Select the appropriate tips for the debridement process based on patient need and access.
4. Set up a powered instrument for periodontal debridement.
5. Using information gathered during the assessment phase, select an appropriate debridement treatment plan for a patient.
6. Determine appropriate treatment codes for a patient who is undergoing periodontal therapy.
7. Assess treatment outcomes based on healing of periodontal structures following treatment.

HOW do I prepare myself to transfer this knowledge to patient care?

 Go to Chapter 31 content on your CD-ROM or search for "Periodontal Therapy" or "Periodontal Tissues."

CD Exercises

- *31-1:Wound Healing:* Order the steps in wound healing.
- *31-2:Wound Healing:* Match rate of healing to each tissue type.
- *31-3: Powered Scaling Instruments—Video:* Match instrument type to hertz and motion of tip.
- *31-4: Tip Design and Applications:* Select the correct tip-to-tooth angle.
- *31-5: Considerations for Use of Powered Instrumentation for Periodontal Debridement:* Determine the appropriate method of debridement for each patient scenario.

- *31-6 to 31-7: Evaluation of Debridement during Procedures—Ann Cronin:* Answer questions based on patient record scenarios for Ann Cronin.
- *31-8 to 31-9: Evaluation of Debridement during Procedures—George Burkett:* Answer questions based on patient record scenarios for George Burkett.
- *31-10: Evaluation of Debridement during Procedures—William Johnston:* Answer questions based on patient record scenarios for William Johnston.
- *31-11 to 31-12: Evaluation of Debridement during Procedures—Adolfo Santana:* Answer questions based on patient record scenarios for Adolfo Santana.

Textbook

Review Case Study 31-1, Therapeutic Selections for the Periodontal Patient, and the case applications.

For important concepts and application of knowledge, review tables, figures, and boxed sections in the textbook.

Tables 31-1 through 31-10 and Box 31-1 may be especially helpful for clinical transfer and may be used as resources:

- Table 31-1: CDT Codes that Correlate with Debridement
- Table 31-2: Risk Factors for Periodontal Disease
- Table 31-3: Bacteria Associated with Periodontal Pathology
- Table 31-4: Page and Schroeder Model for Development of the Periodontal Lesion
- Table 31-5: Healing Rates of Periodontal Tissues
- Table 31-6: Comparison of Characteristics of Powered Instruments
- Table 31-7: Tip Characteristics
- Table 31-8: Tip Selection Guidelines
- Table 31-9: Similarities and Differences between Magnetostrictive and Piezoelectric Instrumentation
- Table 31-10: Debridement for Varying Clinical Conditions
- Box 31-1: Two-Handed Endoscopic Instrumentation Technique

HOW do I perform these skills?

evolve

A printable version of this checklist is available on your Evolve Student Resources.

To complete mechanical debridement procedures successfully, I will:

- ☐ Review health history and prevention survey for considerations prohibiting the use of powered instruments.
- ☐ Select the appropriate instrument tips for periodontal debridement (manual or powered).
- ☐ Discuss with the patient the process of pathogenesis and healing in relationship with the need for periodontal debridement.
- ☐ Prepare unit with appropriate barriers to prevent contamination.
- ☐ Select the appropriate tips for the debridement process based on patient need and access.
- ☐ Use high-volume suction, an aerosol reduction device, or both.
- ☐ Prepare patient with appropriate barriers to prevent contamination.
- ☐ Use appropriate personal protective equipment (PPE) for operator.
- ☐ Perform procedure evaluation.
  - ☐ Set patient expectations (outcomes).
  - ☐ Document findings and procedure in chart.

HOW can I more effectively use this knowledge?

Critical Thinking Activities

Use the following worksheet to complete your activitiy #5.

1. Develop a dialog with Mrs. Cronin to discuss the role of *risk factors* that are relevant in her periodontal disease management and control, specifically the role of diabetes, previous incomplete dental treatment, previous periodontal disease, and crowding.
2. Evaluate several different ultrasonic systems and determine which system you personally would prefer. Provide the rationale for this decision.
3. Compare and contrast the various evaluation techniques and equipment available (explorer, clinical indices, and endoscope) to determine effectiveness of instrumentation with various powered and hand instruments. Consider aspects such as length of time needed to complete the procedure, specific location or site being instrumented, instrument, being used, clinical conditions before instrumentation, and healing response to treatment.

4. With the following patient scenarios, identify and discuss aspects (positive and negative) that will affect periodontal debridement procedures on this patient, then determine an instrumentation sequence that will be most appropriate for each scenario.
   a. Patient with crowded teeth
   b. Patient with full-mouth cosmetic restorations, including implants
   c. Patient with diabetes
   d. Patient with immunosuppressed or immunocompromised health condition
   e. Patient with moderate dental fear
   f. Patient with dentin hypersensitivity
   g. Patient with moderate to deep periodontal pocketing
   h. Patient who has never had his or her teeth cleaned and has moderate to heavy supragingival and subgingival calculus
   i. Patient with light plaque biofilm, no pocketing over 3 mm, and healthy gingival tissue
5. Work in groups of three to evaluate ultrasonic instrumentation setup and patient preparation. One student serves as the clinician, one as the patient, and one as the evaluator. Rotate roles until all students have had the opportunity to serve in all capacities. On Worksheet #1, have the other students enter feedback regarding your actions as a clinician.
6. Ask a classmate to relate specific clinical case scenarios. Determine the appropriate method of periodontal debridement and select the tip or tips to be used in the process.
7. Practice using a powered instrument on an extracted tooth or typodont, and follow the fundamentals for instrumentation.
8. Assist a senior student or a practicing hygienist who is using a powered instrument and perform the following items with him or her:
   a. Help set up and prepare the unit and patient.
   b. Discuss with the operator the rationale for use of the powered instrument and specifics about the case.
   c. Help evacuate water and keep the patient dry. If an aerosol reduction device is available, then place it on the high-velocity evacuation tip and see whether a visible reduction occurs in spray or splatter.
   d. Observe the tip or tips selected for use, and determine the reason for selection.
   e. Observe the fundamentals of instrumentation, and determine whether the operator follows the fundamentals.
9. Role-play with a student partner to provide informed consent to periodontal therapy using powered instruments.

Worksheet #1

Use this form as a feedback mechanism for Critical Thinking Activity #5.

Activity   Feedback

Unit Preparation

Armamentarium is selected and brought to unit.   _____

Water is hooked up.   _____

Electrical source is secured.   _____

Power setting is appropriate.   _____

Water flow is appropriate.   _____

Infection control measures are followed.   _____

Patient Preparation

Patient records are reviewed for contraindications.   _____

Information is given appropriate to patient understanding
and procedure.   _____

Questions are encouraged and answered.   _____

Appropriate draping is applied.   _____

Appropriate infection control protocol is followed.   _____

Tip Selection

Tip selection is appropriate for area and condition.   _____

Tip is applied at appropriate angle to tooth.   _____

Tip is kept in constant motion.   _____

Appropriate water evacuation is followed.   _____

Appropriate infection control protocol is followed.   _____

Unit Breakdown

Armamentarium is prepared for sterilization as
appropriate.   _____

Electrical source is disconnected.   _____

Water hoses are properly drained.   _____

Unit is returned to dispensary or holding area, as applicable. _____

Appropriate infection control protocol is followed.   _____

165

Chapter **31**   **Powered Instrumentation and Periodontal Debridement**

DO I have all the answers?

Review Questions

Check your answers against the Answer Key at the back of this Study Guide to assess what you have learned.

1. Which Current Dental Terminology (CDT) code is used for scaling and root planing?
   a. 1110
   b. 4910
   c. 4341
   d. 4355
   e. 4381

2. When should the current status of self-care and deposit accumulation be evaluated?
   a. At the conclusion of treatment
   b. During treatment
   c. Before periodontal debridement treatment
   d. Only at the initial evaluation

3. Water serves which one of the following purposes when used with a magnetostrictive ultrasonic scaler?
   a. Acts as lavage and coolant
   b. Increases frequency and power
   c. Increases speed and tip vibration
   d. Decreases speed and tip vibration

4. Debridement can include which one of the following procedures?
   a. Brushing and flossing
   b. Polishing
   c. Exploratory stroke with explorer or hand instrument
   d. Scaling and root planing
   e. All of the above

5. Which one of the following conditions has been found to be most virulent?
   a. Adherent plaque biofilm
   b. Imbedded calculus
   c. Burnished calculus
   d. Nonadherent plaque biofilm
   e. Supragingival plaque biofilm

6. Which one of the following etiologic factors of periodontal disease are managed through periodontal debridement?
   a. Dental plaque biofilm and calculus
   b. Immunocompromising systemic diseases
   c. Genetic factors
   d. Tobacco use
   e. Poor nutrition

7. According to the Page and Schroeder model for development of the periodontal lesion, which one of the following lesions histologically has extensive destruction of collagen fibers, a predominance of plasma cells, and regeneration of transseptal fibers?
   a. Initial lesion
   b. Early lesion
   c. Established lesion
   d. Advanced lesion

8. What is the healing rate for gingival surface epithelium?
   a. 5 days
   b. 7 to 10 days
   c. 10 to 14 days
   d. 21 to 28 days
   e. 4 to 6 weeks

9. What are measurable clinical indicators of healing?
   a. Increase in probing depth
   b. Gingival inflammation
   c. Bleeding on probing
   d. High plaque biofilm index
   e. Probing depth reduction

10. What is the action of water that is directed toward the tip and is atomized by the vibration of the tip, creating air cavities in the water?
    a. Magnetostriction
    b. Piezoelectric
    c. Cavitation
    d Sonication

11. Which one of the following are positive effects of ultrasonic and sonic instrumentation?
    a. Removal of stain and irritation of the pulp caused by excess heat generation
    b. Removal of calculus and organization of bacterial colonies
    c. Disruption of bacterial plaque biofilm and removal of calculus

12. The universal standard supragingival tip designed for the magnetostrictive or piezoelectric scaling units can do which one of the following when used correctly?
    a. Successfully debride Class I, II, and III furcations
    b. Remove heavy ledges of calculus
    c. Thoroughly debride the entire mouth of light to moderate subgingival calculus
    d. Debride deep periodontal pockets

13. What is the correct power setting for thin perio-ultrasonic tips?
    a. High power
    b. Low-moderate power
    c. Moderate-high power
    d. Power setting that facilitates deposit removal

14. The purpose of using a 30-second preprocedural mouthrinse with chlorhexidine or Listerine before ultrasonic debridement is to:
    a. Promote tissue healing
    b. Reduce microorganisms in aerosols
    c. Reduce bleeding during instrumentation
    d. Improve mouth odor during instrumentation

15. You are using the ultrasonic scaler with a thin universal insert when the handle starts to get hot. What should you do?
    a. Get another ultrasonic unit.
    b. Discontinue use and use hand instruments.
    c. Remove the tip, fill the handle with water, and reinsert the tip.
    d. Switch the insert tip.
16. Which of the following is characteristic of magnetostrictive ultrasonic technology?
    a. Linear motion
    b. Elliptical motion
    c. Two active sides of the tip
    d. Ceramic discs as an energy source
17. The power knob on an ultrasonic unit controls which of the following?
    a. Length of the stroke
    b. Frequency
    c. Tuning
    d. Water output

WHERE do I go for more information or support?

evolve

For suggested web sites and agencies, additional readings and resources, and more chapter-specific information, please consult your Evolve Student Resources. Because of the ever-changing nature of the Internet, please keep in mind that web sites listed and their content may change.

 CD-ROM

Reference files: As you work through the CD-ROM exercises, you should be able to print reference files and add them to your class materials. No specific reference files apply this chapter.

HOW can I keep track of my progress toward competence?

As an ongoing picture of progress, record and monitor clinical experiences relating to Chapter 31 content in your Portfolio.

Self-Reflection

On a regular basis, review these experiences (with a faculty member). Identify strengths, weaknesses (not just numbers), and changes that you would incorporate into your clinical care plan now that you have had these experiences.

32 Cosmetic and Therapeutic Polishing

WHY do I need to know about Cosmetic and Therapeutic Polishing?

This chapter assists the dental hygiene student in the understanding of dental stains, the professional treatment options available to remove those stains, and the attentiveness necessary to maintain tooth structure and esthetic restorations in the polishing process.

WHAT will I be able to do with this knowledge?

1. Explain to a colleague, patient, or employer the relationship of polishing to the therapeutic and cosmetic goals for oral care.
2. Use cleaning agents rather than polishing agents when clinically appropriate. Select appropriate agents for cleaning and polishing esthetic restorative materials.
3. Classify the various dental stains as either *endogenous* or *exogenous* and be able to determine whether the stain can be removed and, if so, which polishing procedure can remove the stain.
4. Select Porte, engine, or air-powder polishing and the appropriate polishing agent, based on the requirements of the patient's oral condition, his or her response to care, and the equipment and time available.
5. Apply appropriate procedures for each of the polishing methods to remove stains without causing trauma to the oral structures and restorations or discomfort to the patient.
6. Summarize the research findings that suggest the limited therapeutic benefit for coronal polishing and the more relevant therapeutic value of root polishing.
7. Adopt and implement a successful policy of polishing for clinical practice.

HOW do I prepare myself to transfer this knowledge to patient care?

 Go to Chapter 32 content on your CD-ROM or search for "Stain."

CD Exercises

- *32-1: Classification of Dental Stains and Tooth Discoloration:* Understand stain classifications by looking through various intraoral photographs.
- *32-2 and 32-3: Professional Treatment of Extrinsic Stains:* Given a specific patient scenario, select proper polishing methods and agents.

- *32-4 to 32-8: Professional Treatment of Extrinsic Stains:* Review specific patient scenarios (for patients Cronin, Burkett, Johnston, E. Bjork, and Santana) from cases on the CD-ROM and answer polishing questions to help in decision making.

Textbook
Review Case Study 32-1, Selecting the Appropriate Polishing Method, and the case applications. Then consider the following:

- Case Study 32-1 describes a patient with various clinical situations and needs who has requested dental hygiene care. From the information in the chapter, you should be able to evaluate the various situations and determine clinical solutions appropriate to Mr. Smith's needs and requests.
- With the information provided in the chapter and classroom discussion, you should be able to look at any patient and determine appropriate treatment steps regarding stain and polishing.

For important concepts and application of knowledge, review tables, figures, and boxed sections in the textbook.

Tables, boxes, or figures listed here may be especially helpful for clinical transfer and may be used as a clinical resource:

- Box 32-1: Contraindications for Use of Oral Prophylaxis Polishing Paste
- Box 32-2: Principles for Rubber-Cup Polishing
- Figures 32-1 through 32-17 show extrinsic and intrinsic stains in various categories.
- Figures 32-19 through 32-21 show rubber cup polishing.
- Figures 32-25 through 32-27 show air-powder polishing.
- Tables 32-1 through 32-16

HOW do I perform these skills?

evolve

A printable version of this checklist is available on your Evolve Student Resources.

Rubber-Cup Polishing
To perform rubber-cup polishing successfully, I will:

☐ Review patient health history and treatment plan for any contraindications to the procedure.

169

- Obtain necessary equipment: hand piece, prophy angle with specific attachment (brush or cup), dental floss, and disclosing solution.
- Use proper personal protective equipment for patient and operator.
- Use proper operator positioning.
- Use a modified pen grasp.
- Establish a stable fulcrum.
- Identify type of stain.
- Identify areas that should not be polished (e.g., implants).
- Select the least abrasive polishing agent possible that with thoroughly remove plaque biofilm and stain.
- Use proper techniques to reduce unnecessary iatrogenic abrasion on exposed enamel and dentinal surfaces during the procedure.
- Apply polishing agent for correct length of time on a surface.
- Use appropriate speed.
- Use appropriate pressure.
- Thoroughly rinse patient's dentition to remove all residual polishing agents.
- Floss proximal areas with either dental floss or dental tape.
- Inspect for remaining stain with good intraoral light, compressed air, and mouth mirror or disclosing solution.
- Remove any remaining plaque biofilm or stain by reinstrumentation or repolishing the surface.
- Floss interproximal surfaces.
- Set patient expectations (outcomes).

Air-Powder Polishing

To complete air-powder polishing successfully, I will:

- Review patient health history and treatment plan for any contraindications to the procedure.
- Obtain necessary equipment: air-polisher, abrasive powder, floss, disclosing solution, high-speed evacuation system, and preprocedural antimicrobial rinse.
- Use proper personal protective equipment for patient and operator.
- Prepare patient appropriately because of excessive aerosols produced while air-powder polishing.
- Use proper operator positioning.
- Check the amount of water and powder coming from the unit before activation in the patient's mouth.
- Use modified pen grasp.
- Establish a stable fulcrum.
- Use proper tip angulation.

- Apply polishing agent for correct length of time on a surface.
- Use appropriate speed.
- Use appropriate pressure.
- Thoroughly rinse patient's dentition to remove all residual polishing agents.
- Floss proximal areas with either dental floss or dental tape.
- Inspect for remaining stain with good intraoral light, compressed air, and mouth mirror or disclosing solution.
- Remove any remaining plaque biofilm or stain by reinstrumentation or repolishing the surface.
- Floss interproximal surfaces.
- Set patient expectations (outcomes).
- Document findings and procedure in chart.

HOW can I more effectively use this knowledge?

Critical Thinking Activities

Use the following worksheets to complete activities #1 and #9.

1. Develop a treatment plan for Mr. Smith, whose case was presented at the beginning of the chapter. Determine which polishing procedure or combination of procedures would best meet Mr. Smith's clinical and therapeutic goals. Discuss the rationale for each procedure and the specific factors that need to be addressed. Record this information for Mr. Smith as well as for the CD-ROM patients on Worksheet #1.
2. Avoid brushing your teeth for one morning. Rinse your mouth with grape juice, then swallow or expectorate. Describe how your mouth feels and the appearance of your teeth and deposits. Which deposits do you think are stained? How do you think this relates to not brushing after meals and eating colored foods? Why do you "feel" the grape juice remaining in your mouth? Evaluate the ease of removing the stained deposits.
3. Examine several student partners. If intrinsic stains are found, then try to relate them to childhood diseases, medications, fluorides, restorative materials, or other sources. If extrinsic stains are found, then try to identify whether they can be related to tea, coffee, or tobacco consumption (or a combination of these factors).
4. Polish stain from a partner's teeth using a Porte polisher, engine polisher, and air-powder polisher. Compare the results, the effort, and time involved, as well as your partner's preference.
5. Examine the variety of tips available for use in the Porte and engine polishers.
6. Perform routine maintenance on the hand piece and autoclavable prophylaxis angle used for engine polishing in your clinic.

7. Given a nonfunctioning engine polisher, determine why the unit is not working and correct the problem.

8. Evaluate the effectiveness and quality of disposable prophylaxis angles after clinical application of each.

9. Use the air-powder polisher to polish a quadrant of teeth that are heavily stained. Polish a second quadrant with an engine-driven rubber cup. Compare the results in terms of (1) cleanliness of the teeth, (2) time, (3) patient acceptance, and (4) amount of recurrent stain remaining after polishing, at the recall visit, or both. Record these results on Worksheet #2.

10. Take two pennies and draw a line to divide each in half. On one half apply dry pumice with a rubber cup. On the other half apply dry chalk with a second rubber cup. Examine each for scratches. On the second penny, apply a slurry of pumice with a rubber cup to one half and a slurry of chalk with a new rubber cup to the other half. Examine each for differences in smoothness and luster. The same exercise can be performed with any abrasive or polishing method.

Worksheet #1

Record your evaluation from Critical Thinking Activity #1 on the following form, then continue by selecting the appropriate polishing method and agents for each of the patients on the CD-ROM.

Patient Name	Polishing Method of Choice	Polishing Agents	Rationale for Selections
Bill Smith			
Ann Cronin			
William Johnston			
George Burkett			
Maria Bjork			
Eva Bjork			
Subra Mani			
Elena Guri			
Adolfo Santana			

Worksheet #2

Record your findings from Critical Thinking Activity #9 on the following worksheet.

Air-Powder Polisher	Engine-Driven Rubber Cup Polisher with Fine Prophy Paste	Engine-Driven Rubber Cup Polisher with Coarse Prophy Paste	Toothbrush and Toothpaste
Cleanliness of the teeth			
Time spent to clean the teeth			
Patient acceptance of treatment.			
Amount of recurrent stain remaining after polishing			

173

DO I have all the answers?

Review Questions

Check your answers against the Answer Key at the back of this Study Guide to assess what you have learned. Questions 1 through 3 refer to Case Study 32-1.

1. Which of the following polishing procedures is (are) indicated in the polishing of Mr. Smith's teeth?
   a. Air-powder polisher
   b. Coarse prophylaxis paste with engine polisher
   c. Diamond polishing paste
   d. All of the above

2. Which of the following polishing procedures should be performed first on Mr. Smith?
   a. Use of an air-powder polisher
   b. Use of a coarse prophylaxis paste with engine polisher
   c. Use of a diamond polishing paste

3. Which of the following phrases describes Mr. Smith's stain classification?
   a. Environmental exogenous
   b. Environmental endogenous
   c. Developmental endogenous

4. Which of the following health concerns contraindicates use of air-powder polishing?
   a. Diabetes
   b. Mitral valve prolapse
   c. Asthma
   d. Chronic migraines

5. Which of the following is the stain classification for a green stain?
   a. Exogenous, extrinsic
   b. Endogenous, intrinsic
   c. Endogenous, extrinsic
   d. Exogenous, intrinsic

6. Which of the following factors affect the abrasiveness of a polishing agent?
   a. Particle size and shape
   b. Particle hardness and concentration
   c. Amount of water and fluoride
   d. Both *a* and *b*
   e. Both *a* and *c*

7. Through which of the following methods can frictional heat be minimized during engine polishing?
   a. Increase the engine speed.
   b. Reduce the engine speed.
   c. Decrease the amount of paste or abrasive.
   d. Increase the amount of time spent on each surface.

8. Which of the following is considered a disadvantage of the Porte polisher?
   a. Portability of unit
   b. Generation of minimal frictional heat
   c. Slow, tedious process
   d. Minimal aerosols produced

9. Which of the following effects does polishing of unexposed root surfaces during a surgical procedure have on disease?
   a. Cosmetic effect
   b. Therapeutic effect
   c. Placebo effect

WHERE do I go for more information or support?

evolve

For suggested web sites and agencies, additional readings and resources, and more chapter-specific information, please consult your Evolve Student Resources. Because of the ever-changing nature of the Internet, please keep in mind that web sites listed and their content may change.

CD-ROM

Reference files: As you work through the CD-ROM exercises, you should be able to print reference files and add them to your class materials. No specific reference files apply to this chapter.

HOW can I keep track of my progress toward competence?

As an ongoing picture of progress, record and monitor clinical experiences relating to Chapter 32 content in your Portfolio.

Self-Reflection

On a regular basis, review these experiences (with a faculty member). Identify strengths, weaknesses (not just numbers), and changes that you would incorporate into your clinical care plan now that you have had these experiences.

33 Dentinal Hypersensitivity

WHY do I need to know about Dentinal Hypersensitivity?

One of the most common, yet misunderstood, challenges within the dental office is dentinal hypersensitivity. A myriad of over-the-counter (OTC) home care products (as well as professionally applied, in-office treatment options) is available to the dental hygienist to recommend and use for this condition. Understanding the various functions and applications of each product and treatment option is essential to make effective clinical decisions.

WHAT will I be able to do with this knowledge?

1. Understand the hydrodynamic theory of pain conduction.
2. Describe the three main categories of stimuli that elicit a pain response and give examples of each.
3. Describe desensitizing agents and products available for self-care.
4. Select office procedures for the treatment of hypersensitivity based on patient needs and evaluate the response to agents.
5. Evaluate the literature on desensitizing agents to determine the most effective products for self-care and professional use.

HOW do I prepare myself to transfer this knowledge to patient care?

 Go to Chapter 33 content on your CD-ROM or search for "Dentinal Hypersensitivity."

CD Exercises

- *33-1: Terminology:* Demonstration of theories of dentinal hypersensitivity and identification of terminology.
- *32-2: Management Strategies for Dentinal Hypersensitivity:* Select decision points for the management of dentinal sensitivity that can be transferred to the reference file.
- *33-3 to 33-6: Administration of Treatment:* Review patients Cronin and Burkett from the CD-ROM.

Textbook
Review Case Study 33-1, Treatment of Dentinal Hypersensitivity to Cold Stimuli, and the case applications.

HOW do I perform these skills?

evolve

A printable version of this checklist is available on your Evolve Student Resources.
To apply a desensitizing agent correctly, I will be able to:

- ☐ Review health history for contraindication to procedure.
- ☐ Obtain patient consent following explanation of procedure.
- ☐ Gather necessary armamentarium.
- ☐ Identify one or more tooth surfaces to be treated.
- ☐ Isolate one or more tooth surfaces to be treated.
- ☐ Gently dry one or more tooth surfaces to be treated (or follow manufacturer's directions for application of agent).
- ☐ Apply desensitizing agent, according to manufacturer's instructions.
- ☐ At treatment completion, gently rinse area.
- ☐ Set patient expectations (outcomes).
- ☐ Document findings and procedure in chart.

HOW can I more effectively use this knowledge?

Critical Thinking Activities
Use the following worksheet to complete activity #2.
1. Determine whether classmates have areas of gingival recession or tooth hypersensitivity.
   a. Test both areas with the following: ice, a blast of air, cold water, hot water, a sharp probe.
   b. What is the most severe reaction in terms of speed of reaction and pain?
   c. Do areas of recession and hypersensitivity differ? If so, why?
   d. What parameters do you think would be best for testing a new antisensitivity agent?
2. Review two publications on desensitizing products, published before and after 1990. Using Worksheet #1, comment on the occurrence of the placebo effect and on the measurements used.

Worksheet #1

After completing Critical Thinking Activity #2, use this form to review one dentifrice and one additional type of desensitizing therapy.

OVERVIEW

Article title _____

Author(s) _____

Publication title _____

Date, volume, issue, page _____

Stated purpose of the study _____

What was being evaluated? _____

METHODOLOGY

Study Design

Was the study design clearly described and appropriate for the investigation? _____

_____

Was the study design double blind? _____

_____

Was the study design single blind? _____

_____

Was the length of investigation sufficient to study the subject? _____

_____

Was interexaminer and intraexaminer reliability stated? _____

_____

Subjects

Was the sample size large enough? _____

_____

Composition of the sample population: Was it appropriate to the therapy used? _____

_____

How many subjects dropped out of the study (through attrition)? _____

_____

Did the researchers attempt to balance the groups? _____

_____

177

DO I have all the answers?

Review Questions

Check your answers against the Answer Key at the back of this Study Guide to assess what you have learned.

1. Which of the following areas of the tooth are considered most sensitive to various stimuli?
   a. Occlusal, incisal
   b. Cervical, proximal
   c. Lingual, cervical
   d. Facial, cervical

2. Dentinal hypersensitivity is a multifactorial condition. Stimuli of a thermal, tactile, chemical, or osmotic nature can result in pain.
   a. The first statement is true; the second is false.
   b. The first statement is false; the second is true.
   c. Both statements are true.
   d. Both statements are false.

3. Desensitizing agents primarily work by which one of the following ways?
   a. Occluding the dentinal tubules
   b. Changing the surface ions
   c. Interfering with neurologic responses
   d. Inhibiting the osmotic pressure between membranes

4. When testing dentin hypersensitivity, the hygienist should perform a differential diagnosis, because without this process, one might make an error in the diagnosis. Which one of the following statements best describes the nature of the previous statement?
   a. The first part of the statement is true; the second is false.
   b. Both parts of the statement are true.
   c. Both parts of the statement are false.
   d. The first part of the statement is false; the second part is true.

5. How does burnishing reduce dentin hypersensitivity?
   a. It removes a smear layer, allowing the dentinal tubules to expand.
   b. It produces a smear layer and occludes the dentinal tubules.
   c. Burnishing alone does not reduce dentin hypersensitivity.
   d. Burnishing is not used to reduce dentin hypersensitivity.

6. Which of the following agents provides the most benefit in reducing dentin hypersensitivity?
   a. Oxalates
   b. Strontium chloride
   c. Potassium nitrate
   d. Fluoride

WHERE do I go for more information or support?

evolve

For suggested web sites and agencies, additional readings and resources, and more chapter-specific information, please consult your Evolve Student Resources. Because of the ever-changing nature of the Internet, please keep in mind that web sites listed and their content may change.

 CD-ROM

Reference files: As you work through the CD-ROM exercises, you should be able to print reference files and add them to your class materials. One exercise for Chapter 33, Management of Dentinal Sensitivity, should be written to a reference file once you have completed it.

HOW can I keep track of my progress toward competence?

As an ongoing picture of progress, record and monitor clinical experiences relating to Chapter 33 content in your Portfolio.

Self-Reflection

On a regular basis, review these experiences (with a faculty member). Identify strengths, weaknesses (not just numbers), and changes that you would incorporate into your clinical care plan now that you have had these experiences.

34 Periodontal Dressings and Suturing

WHY do I need to know about Periodontal Dressings and Suturing?

Dental hygienists seldom have an opportunity to place sutures, but they may have the need to remove sutures, to place and remove periodontal dressings, and to provide postoperative instructions to patients. With the knowledge of wound healing and dental materials, the dental hygienist is in a position to provide patients with an understanding of expectations after surgery and to assess surgical sites when dressings and sutures are removed.

WHAT will I be able to do with this knowledge?

1. Understand the basic concepts of suture materials, suture design, and suturing techniques.
2. List the available periodontal dressings, and state the rationale for their use.
3. Describe the characteristics of the ideal suture material and the ideal periodontal dressing.
4. Discuss the uses, advantages, and limitations of suture materials and periodontal dressings.
5. Assist healthcare professionals in the selection, use, and removal of periodontal sutures and dressings, and explain the use of these materials to patients.

HOW do I prepare myself to transfer this knowledge to patient care?

 Go to Chapter 34 content on your CD-ROM or search for "Sutures."

CD Exercises

- *34-1: Suture Materials:* Match the term to its description.
- *34-2: Suture Removal:* Place suture removal steps in the correct order.
- *34-3: Suture Removal—Ann Cronin:* Order the steps in removal of patient Ann Cronin's sutures.

Textbook

Review Case Study 34-1, Suturing: Three Specific Procedures, which will help you understand the different suture techniques and materials used in each. After reading the chapter and the case applications, consider the following:

- Discuss rationale for the type of sutures used in each case and identify what type of suture material is most likely used for each.

- Describe the technique of surgical dressing placement and provide rationale for treatment choice of using surgical dressing versus periodontal dressing.

For important concepts and application of knowledge, review tables, figures, and boxed sections in the text.

The following elements may be especially helpful for clinical transfer and may be used as clinical resources:

- Box 34-1: Common Suture Materials
- Box 34-2: Characteristics of the Ideal Suture Material
- Box 34-3: Postoperative Care and Procedures
- Box 34-4: Ideal Properties of a Periodontal Dressing
- Figures 34-13 through 13-24 are images of various suture techniques and periodontal dressings.

HOW do I perform these skills?

evolve

A printable version of this checklist is available on your Evolve Student Resources.

To remove periodontal dressing properly, I will:

- Gently dislodge the dressing from the surgical area.
- Clean surgical site.
- Give postoperative instructions.

To remove sutures properly, I will:

- Irrigate the surgical site with an antimicrobial agent.
- Remove remaining periodontal dressing, if applicable.
- Cut sutures.
- Remove sutures.

HOW can I more effectively use this knowledge?

Critical Thinking Activities

1. Manipulate several different types of suture materials, and compare their characteristics, sizes, and handling abilities.
2. Visit a periodontal office, and observe the placement and removal of periodontal sutures and dressings.
3. Practice placing and removing various periodontal sutures and dressings using a model, animal jaw (e.g., pig), or other object (e.g., hot dog).

179

4. Discuss the knowledge acquired in this chapter with fellow students, and paraphrase or restate in your own words the information that is critical to your own practice philosophy.
5. Create several types of cases, and compare the advantages and disadvantages of different suture materials and periodontal dressings under each set of circumstances.

DO I have all the answers?

Review Questions

Check your answers against the Answer Key at the back of this Study Guide to assess what you have learned. Questions 2 and 7 refer to Case Study 34-1.

1. Which one of the following is an example of an absorbable suture material?
   a. Silk
   b. Polypropylene
   c. Nylon
   d. Gut
2. Which suture material was used to support Mr. Augsberger's soft tissue graft?
   a. Chromic gut
   b. Plain gut
   c. Silk
   d. Nylon
3. Which one of the following is the most commonly used suture material in dentistry?
   a. Chromic gut
   b. Silk
   c. Plain gut
   d. Polyester
4. Which one of the following is (are) characteristics of an ideal suture material?
   a. Inhibits bacterial growth
   b. Has a small diameter but great strength
   c. Is comfortable to use and easy to manipulate
   d. Is sterile and conveniently packaged
   e. All of the above
5. Are modern periodontal dressings usually formulated without eugenol?
   a. Yes
   b. No
6. Which one of the following is (are) characteristics of the ideal periodontal dressing?
   a. Sets slowly enough to allow easy manipulation
   b. Maintains its flexibility to prevent easy fracture and withstands distortion
   c. Has an acceptable taste
   d. All of the above
7. Which one of the following types of suturing technique was used for Mrs. Martinez?
   a. Continuous interlocking suture
   b. Simple interrupted loop suture
   c. Continuous double-sling suture
   d. Periosteal suture

WHERE do I go for more information or support?

evolve

For suggested web sites and agencies, additional readings and resources, and more chapter-specific information, please consult your Evolve Student Resources. Because of the ever-changing nature of the Internet, please keep in mind that web sites listed and their content may change.

CD-ROM

Reference files: As you work through the CD-ROM exercises, you should be able to print reference files and add them to your class materials. No specific reference files apply to this chapter.

HOW can I keep track of my progress toward competence?

As an ongoing picture of progress, record and monitor clinical experiences relating to Chapter 34 content in your Portfolio.

Self-Reflection

On a regular basis, review these experiences (with a faculty member). Identify strengths, weaknesses (not just numbers), and changes that you would incorporate into your clinical care plan now that you have had these experiences.

35 Operative Procedures

WHY do I need to know about Operative Procedures?

The dental hygienist can perform simple operative dentistry procedures in selected states within the United States, as well as in other countries around the world. As access to care needs expand in the future, the dental hygienist may play an important role in performing operative dentistry procedures in certain situations. In addition, patients often rely on the dental hygienist to answer questions regarding operative procedures. Every dental hygienist must have an understanding of operative dentistry and how to assist the patient in understanding his or her treatment needs.

WHAT will I be able to do with this knowledge?

1. Assess the patient's needs for operative dental treatment.
2. Discuss the rationale for treatment planning.
3. Describe the characteristics of Classes I through VI cavity preparations.
4. Identify walls, cavosurfaces, line angles, and point angles.
5. Discuss the rationale for minimally invasive treatment.
6. Know the rationale and describe the proper technique for placement of a rubber dam.
7. Discuss the advances in esthetic materials and techniques.
8. Discuss the rationale for use of bases and liners.
9. Compare the advantages and disadvantages of various restorative materials.
10. Describe the function and placement of a matrix.

HOW do I prepare myself to transfer this knowledge to patient care?

 Go to Chapter 35 content on your CD-ROM or search for "Restorative Dentistry."

CD Exercises
- *35-1: Black's Restorative Lesion Classification:* Identify each classification in the GV Black classification system.
- *35-2: Components of Prepared Cavities:* Name cavity preparation walls and angles.
- *35-3: Amalgam or Direct Resin Composite Restorations:* Determine the advantages and disadvantages to the restorative materials of composite and amalgam.

- *35-4: Assess Restorative Needs—Eva Bjork:* Based on patient records and scenarios, assess restorative needs for patient, Eva Bjork.

Textbook
Review Case Study 35-1, Application of Operative Therapies, and the case applications. After reading the case applications in the chapter, consider the following:
- Describe minimally invasive options that might be applied to the patient in this case.
- What type of education or information is necessary to make Mrs. Dixon aware of esthetic interventions for the treatment of her dentition?
- Included in Mrs. Dixon's treatment plan was the need to replace one of the existing Class II amalgam restorations on tooth #19. A matrix system will need to be used in this treatment. Review the matrix system setup, and describe the various matrix materials available and why a matrix system is needed for this type of restoration.
- How would you explain the importance and process of acid-etch, shade selection, and rubber dam to Mrs. Dixon?

For important concepts and application of knowledge, review tables, figures, and boxed sections in the textbook.

The following may be especially helpful for clinical transfer and may be used as a clinical resource:
- Box 35-1: Steps for Clamp Placement
- Box 35-2: Steps for Application of Gingival Retractor Clamp for Class V Restorations
- Box 35-3: Amalgam Placement for Classes I, V, and VI Preparations
- Box 35-4: Amalgam Placement for Class II Preparations

HOW do I perform these skills?

evolve

A printable version of this checklist is available on your Evolve Student Resources.
To place a rubber dam properly, I will:
- ☐ Select proper armamentarium.
- ☐ Identify area for isolation.
- ☐ Select proper rubber dam holder.
- ☐ Select proper rubber dam material.
- ☐ Explain treatment to patient.

181

□ Select proper rubber dam clamp.

□ Ligate rubber dam clamp.

□ Punch rubber dam holes according to tooth location, size, shape and size of arch, position and spacing of teeth, and type of preparation.

□ Lubricate patient's lips.

□ Place powdered side of the dam facing the clinician.

□ Properly place the rubber dam onto clamp (winged or wingless).

□ Tuck the dam into the sulcus around each tooth to prevent seepage of sulcular fluid and saliva.

□ Stabilize the rubber dam by ligating a piece of dental floss around the most anterior tooth or by wedging a small piece of rubber into the embrasure between the last exposed tooth and the rubber dam.

□ Insert saliva ejector under the rubber dam onto the line of floor of the mouth.

To remove a rubber dam properly, I will:

□ Use high-volume evacuation to remove all debris from the operating field.

□ Remove a gingival retractor, if used.

□ Remove the ligature or rubber dam wedge from the most anterior tooth.

□ Stretch the facial aspect of the dam away from the teeth.

□ Place one finger under the stretched dam while cutting the interdental areas of the dam.

□ Cut the entire septum with one stroke from the facial aspect.

□ Pull the dam in a lingual direction.

□ Check that dam appears as it did before placement.

□ Rinse and evacuate oral cavity.

□ Examine the soft tissue for any trauma.

□ Set patient expectations (outcomes).

□ Document findings and procedure in chart.

HOW can I more effectively use this knowledge?

Critical Thinking Activities

1. Form a study group and research the differences in the practice patterns of operative therapies among the various states.

2. Discuss the differences in practice patterns with your instructors, especially those who have practiced in various states.

3. Conduct a panel discussion with dental hygienists who practice in both traditional and expanded-function settings to learn about the associated challenges.

4. Obtain prepared dentoforms.

   a. Identify cavosurface margins, point angles, line angles, walls, and floors.

b. Practice the placement of various matrix systems.

c. Practice the placement of the rubber dam in various areas of the dentoform.

d. Practice the placement and finishing of various restorative materials.

5. Evaluate a classmate's restorations and request that he or she critique your restorations.

DO I have all the answers?

Review Questions

Check your answers against the Answer Key at the back of this Study Guide to assess what you have learned.

1. Which one of the following statements best describes the differences between a Class I cavity preparation and a Class II cavity preparation?

   a. Class II includes the extension of a Class I into the incisal edge of an anterior tooth.

   b. Class II includes the extension of a Class I into the facial or lingual gingival margin area.

   c. Class II includes the extension of a Class I into the proximal area over the marginal ridge.

   d. Class II includes the extension of a Class I and is located on a cusp tip.

2. All of the following are advantages to minimally invasive dentistry *except* which one?

   a. Preserves tooth structure

   b. Increases tooth resistance to further breakdown

   c. Requires extension of preparation for prevention

   d. Uses less amalgam

3. Which of the following lists describes the major components found in dental amalgam?

   a. Silver, tin, mercury

   b. Silver, nickel, tin

   c. Silver, copper, zinc

   d. Silver, mercury, gold

4. Resin composite is a tooth-colored restoration, resulting in less marginal leakage than amalgam.

   a. Both the first and the second parts of the statement are true.

   b. The first part of the statement is true; the second part is false.

   c. The first part of the statement is false; the second part is true.

   d. Both the first and the second parts of the statement are false.

5. Which one of the following reasons best describes why a dental practitioner would use a wooden wedge?

   a. Increases setting time and hardness of amalgam

   b. Prevents overhang and allows for easier removal of the matrix band

   c. Decreases amalgam setting time and assists with occlusal adjustment

   d. Increases amalgam setting time and prevents overhang

WHERE do I go for more information or support?

evolve

For suggested web sites and agencies, additional readings and resources, and more chapter-specific information, please consult your Evolve Student Resources. Because of the ever-changing nature of the Internet, please keep in mind that web sites listed and their content may change.

CD-ROM

Reference files: As you work through the CD-ROM exercises, you should be able to print reference files and add them to your class materials. No specific reference files apply to this chapter.

HOW can I keep track of my progress toward competence?

As an ongoing picture of progress, record and monitor clinical experiences relating to Chapter 35 content in your Portfolio.

Self-Reflection

On a regular basis, review these experiences (with a faculty member). Identify strengths, weaknesses (not just numbers), and changes that you would incorporate into your clinical care plan now that you have had these experiences.

36 Esthetics

WHY do I need to know about Esthetics?

Dental hygienists need only consider the driving forces of the population demographics, advances in material science and technologies, and pop culture trends such as makeover television programs to understand the esthetic revolution. Esthetic dentistry and whitening is now synonymous with patients who desire not only healthy mouths but also attractive smiles. Getting involved in esthetic and whitening services increases a dental hygienists' value to the dental office team. Many dental hygienists take on the role of in-office whitening coordinator, developing restorative maintenance programs or becoming patient advocates for restorative home care regimens. Esthetics and whitening are challenging ways to expand dental hygienists' careers and bring new dimensions to their diagnostic skills.

WHAT will I be able to do with this knowledge?

1. Discuss the validation of the psychologic and sociologic effects of physical attractiveness on human self-esteem.
2. Generate an understanding of esthetic dentistry and dental hygiene and its value to dental hygienists and their patients.
3. Establish a process for designing effective "smile assessments."
4. Review evidence-based dental and dental hygiene techniques that preserve a patient's restored smile while maintaining oral health.
5. Discuss methods of identifying and documenting esthetic restorations, preventive maintenance, and home care solutions that are currently available.
6. Select appropriate professional supportive care measures and recommend home self-care techniques for various esthetic restorations.
7. Assist the patient in understanding the importance of his or her role in preserving and maintaining restorative dentistry and oral health.
8. Assist the patient in becoming proficient in maintaining healthy gingival tissue, emphasizing the importance of daily dental plaque biofilm elimination and commitment to supportive care.
9. List tolerability issues regarding the use of tooth-whitening agents that contain peroxide.
10. Discuss the advantages, disadvantages, clinical indications, and contraindications for tooth whitening.

11. List the common side effects of dental whitening and their contributing factors.
12. Explain the importance of dental professional and patient communication throughout the bleaching process, as well as the role of the dental hygienist in dental-whitening therapy.
13. Demonstrate and describe the clinical techniques used for fabrication of a night guard.
14. Compare and contrast the whitening effect of in-office and home-applied vital tooth bleaching and how these two systems might be used in conjunction with one another.
15. Discuss the effects of whitening agents on enamel, dentin, pulp, and restorative materials.
16. Investigate products currently available for cosmetic whitening, including professional, over-the-counter, in-office, and home-applied whiteners.
17. Describe the role of dental hygienists in planning, implementing, and evaluating cosmetic-whitening procedures.

HOW do I prepare myself to transfer this knowledge to patient care?

 Go to Chapter 36 content on your CD-ROM or search for "Esthetic Dentistry."

CD Exercises

- *36-1: Evolution of Bleaching:* Dispel the myths about whitening procedures through a series of true-false questions.
- *36-2 to 36-5: Patient Selection: Indications and Contraindications:* Assess the esthetic needs of several patient cases and make recommendations for tooth whitening.

Textbook

Review the case studies and several case applications.

For important concepts and application knowledge, the following tables, boxes, or figures may be especially helpful for clinical transfer and may be used as a clinical resource:

- Table 36-1: Comparison of Available Polishing Products
- Table 36-2: Shade Guide Selection and Setup
- Figure 36-7: Value-oriented Vita shade guide.
- Box 36-1: Reasons for Maintaining Esthetic Restorations

- Box 36-3: Hygiene Occlusal Analysis and Clinical Signs: Observe and Record Standards and Deviations
- Box 36-4: Technique Guide for Polishing Esthetic Restorations
- Box 36-5: Self-Care of Esthetic Restorations

HOW do I perform these skills?

evolve

A printable version of this checklist is available on your Evolve Student Resources.

To polish esthetic restorations properly, I will:

Step 1: Identify

- ☐ Identify the difference between natural tooth structure and the type of restorations.

Step 2: Evaluate

- ☐ Determine the extent of polishing necessary—renewing or replacement.

Step 3: Complete Polishing Procedure

- ☐ Complete plaque biofilm or light stain removal.
- ☐ Complete medium to heavy stain removal.
  - ☐ Begin to polish with extra-fine composite paste in a wet environment.
  - ☐ Distribute polish adequately over the entire surface and use a light intermittent stroke contacting the restorative or tooth surface for no more than 15 to 30 seconds each. (The goal is for restoration polishing, not recontouring or margin obliteration.)
  - ☐ Carry paste interproximally with floss, and rinse to clear area before reexamining.

Step 4: Re-Evaluate

If stain removal and high shine, leaving the desired surface texture on, is the goal, and if a paste alone did not achieve the desired results, then it may be necessary to move on to more aggressive techniques.

- ☐ Once stain removal is achieved, reverse the process and finish polishing with the least abrasive composite polish or instrument to achieve the desired high shine and surface texture.
- ☐ Complete interproximal stain removal with aluminum oxide polishing strips.

Step 5: Review Composites

Remember if stain at the margins is present:

- *State practice acts and allowable functions will determine the choice of instrumentation for this step.*
- *Severe microleakage or open margins may require restoration replacement and a physician's evaluation.*
  - ☐ Start with either a coarse point, diamond-impregnated rubber polishing points, slow-speed hand piece with a polishing or finishing bur, air abrasion (aluminum oxide), or high-speed device (carbide finishing bur, fissure prep bur).

- ☐ Gently roughen the restoration to minimally open the margins, and remove the irregular marginal staining and/or *black line*.
- ☐ Once the marginal stain is removed, scrub area clean by using a mixture of a cleaner or disinfectant and pumice with a brush applicator, or use a chlorhexidine antibacterial scrub and a bristle brush in a slow-speed hand piece.
- ☐ Wash and dry the area.
- ☐ Etch the discrepancy several millimeters past the previously stained area. Use a disposable brush or applicator tip to agitate the etchant for 15 to 20 seconds. When renewing a composite restoration, the clinician may choose to use a plastic strip or guard interproximally to preserve the adjacent tooth.
- ☐ Rinse off the etchant for 5 seconds with an air-water spray.
- ☐ Apply enamel-bonding agent, following the manufacturer's directions.
- ☐ Apply the *composite material*. A sable brush, small soft paintbrush, or applicator brush can be used to manipulate the renewal sealant.
- ☐ Cure for 40 seconds.
- ☐ Remove Mylar strip or guard if used.
- ☐ Smooth or polish area with composite polishing paste.

Step 6: Increase Vitality and Longevity

Once either the stain removal procedures or the renewal services are complete, I will follow the final steps to further preserve the integrity of the restoration:

- ☐ Following polishing the renewed restoration and enamel, use a disposable brush or applicator tip to agitate the etchant for 5 seconds. When applying a composite sealant, the clinician may choose to use a plastic strip or guard interproximally to preserve the adjacent tooth.
- ☐ Rinse off the etchant for 5 seconds with an air-water spray.
- ☐ Dry.
- ☐ Apply a composite surface sealant vigorously into the entire restoration, including margins, with a mini-brush tip.
- ☐ Gently blow off any excess.
- ☐ Cure the composite surface sealant for 20 seconds.
- ☐ Administer a tray with a neutral sodium fluoride application.

HOW can I more effectively use this knowledge?

Critical Thinking Activities

Use the following worksheet provided to complete activity #1.

1. Audit approximately 12 patient charts. Then schedule an informal learning session with a restorative dentist, and ask questions concerning restorative treatment plans. Record answers on Worksheet #1. Questions may include the following:

- What role does occlusion play in determining restorative materials?
- How large does an old restoration have to get before you would decide to place a veneer or crown?
- What conditions could be esthetically corrected with composite materials, indirect restorations, bleaching, cosmetic contouring, and so on?

2. Soak a variety of prefabricated teeth in chromogenic liquids. Next polish the teeth with a variety of polishing agents, and evaluate the surface texture of the materials and natural teeth.
3. Schedule visits to a local cosmetic dental office and dental laboratory. Take a tour, observe the fabrication of indirect restorations, and/or observe an esthetic assessment or restorative procedure.
4. Set up the shade guide from lightest to darkest. Take turns with your classmates and hold the shade guide so that you and your classmates can see the colors. Practice selecting and recording the appropriate shade for an anterior incisor, maxillary canine, and posterior tooth.
5. With the help of a classmate, obtain, pour, and trim alginate impressions.
6. Fabricate a nightguard vital bleaching (NVB) tray for the maxillary arch with the following specifications:
   Right quadrant: nonreservoir, nonscalloped
   Left quadrant: reservoir, scalloped
7. Evaluate a patient's health history and clinical assessment to determine whether cosmetic whitening is warranted.
8. Debate the advantages and disadvantages of tray (NVB) versus OTC bleaching systems.
9. With the use of a tooth shade guide system, evaluate the clinical results of cosmetic whitening on a patient who has completed the procedure.
10. Peruse the Internet for evidence-based studies on esthetic materials and whitening agents (www.medline.com).

Worksheet #1

Use this worksheet to record responses from your interview with the dentist in Critical Thinking Activity #1.

Question	Dentist Interviewed
What role does occlusion play in determining restorative materials?	
How large does an old restoration have to get before you would decide to place a veneer or crown?	
What conditions might be esthetically corrected with composite materials?	
What conditions might be esthetically corrected with indirect restorations?	
What conditions might be esthetically corrected with bleaching?	
What conditions might be esthetically corrected with cosmetic contouring?	
What additional cosmetic-type procedures are performed in this practice?	

188

DO I have all the answers?

Review Questions

Check your answers agianst the Answer Key at the back of this Study Guide to assess what you have learned. Questions 17 to 23 refer to the case studies presented in the chapter.

1. Composite bonding is indicated for restoring which of the following?
   a. Small to moderate carious lesions or defects
   b. Anterior and posterior teeth
   c. Abrasion or erosion defects that cause wear near the gum line
   d. All of the above

2. Which one of the following choices best describes the advantages of composite resins?
   a. Limited durability
   b. Excellent esthetics and conservative treatment options
   c. Sensitive techniques
   d. Subject to staining, wear, or chipping over time

3. Resin composite restorations are subject to softening by which one of the following professional and self-care product ingredients?
   a. Mint flavoring
   b. 1.1% sodium mouthwash
   c. Acidulated phosphate fluoride
   d. Water

4. Which of the following are general guidelines that dental hygienists should consider when assessing esthetic treatment options?
   a. Material selection, restoration, fabrication.
   b. Restorative clinician's expertise.
   c. Both *a* and *b* are correct.
   d. Neither choice is corrcct.

5. Dental hygienists need which of the following group of armamentarium to assist in the identification and recording of esthetic materials?
   a. Small surgical air tip, mirror, high-speed hand piece
   b. Radiographs, digital images, study model
   c. Small surgical air tip, magnification loupe, trans-illumination
   d. Radiographs, bite registration, impressions

6. Protecting the definitive restoration from parafunctional habits can be achieved by recommending which one of the following postoperative appliances?
   a. Orthodontic removable retainer
   b. Night guard
   c. Sports mouthguard
   d. Palatal expander

7. Traditional prophylactic paste can be safety used on which one of the following restorative materials?
   a. Acrylic
   b. Ceramic
   c. Gold
   d. Composites

8. Which one of the following home-applied bleaching concentrations is safe and effective, as determined by the American Dental Association (ADA)?
   a. 5% hydrogen peroxide (H_2O_2)
   b. 10% carbamide peroxide
   c. 15% carbamide peroxide
   d. 10% to 15% H_2O_2

9. Which one of the following tray designs is recommended for patients who experience gingival irritation from the bleaching gel?
   a. Reservoir
   b. Scalloped
   c. Nonreservoir
   d. Rigid

10. In-office professional bleaching offers which of the following advantages?
    a. Less monitoring during the procedure
    b. Faster whitening results
    c. Lower concentration of hydrogen peroxide
    d. All of the above

11. In saliva, carbamide peroxide is converted into which one of the following substances?
    a. Potassium nitrate
    b. Glycerin
    c. Carbopol
    d. H_2O_2

12. Which one of the following is a disadvantage of the use of whitening strips for vital tooth bleaching?
    a. Less tooth coverage
    b. Cost
    c. Difficult to use
    d. Uncomfortable tray

13. Proxigel was first used for dental bleaching, but because of its _____, it was replaced by _____ gels specific for dental bleaching.
    a. Poor substantivity; less viscous
    b. High concentration; more fluidlike
    c. Poor substantivity, more viscous
    d. High concentration; less fluidlike

14. Which one of the following conditions is a side effect of cosmetic whitening?
    a. Carcinogenicity
    b. Genotoxicity
    c. Pulpal necrosis
    d. Gingival irritation

15. When is the most appropriate time to provide realistic expectations of cosmetic whitening to the patient?
    a. After treatment is completed
    b. Before and after treatment
    c. Before, during, and after treatment
    d. Before cosmetic whitening is begun

16. Tooth sensitivity associated with dentist-prescribed home-applied bleaching can be controlled and reduced through which of the following methods?
    a. Reducing the frequency of bleaching
    b. Reducing bleaching time
    c. Using a lower concentration of carbamide peroxide
    d. All of the above

17. Which one of the following is the *most likely* cause for the brown discoloration noted on Jimmy's maxillary incisor?
    a. Disturbance in enamel-dentin matrix
    b. Ingestion of high levels of fluoride
    c. History of trauma
    d. Interruption of permanent tooth formation
18. Which one of the following tray designs would be indicated for Jimmy?
    a. Scalloped, reservoir
    b. Scalloped, nonreservoir
    c. Nonscalloped, reservoir
    d. Nonscalloped, nonreservoir
19. Which one of the following degrees of tetracycline (TCN) stain does Ms. O'Bryan most likely exhibit?
    a. First
    b. Second
    c. Third
    d. Fourth
20. The tray design was changed at Ms. O'Bryan's 7-month recall for which one of the following reasons?
    a. To obtain cervical third coverage
    b. Because Ms. O'Bryan misplaced her original tray
    c. Because the original tray was ill fitting
    d. Because the bleaching material was changed
21. After successful bleaching therapy, which of the following best represents the next phase of treatment?
    a. Routine prophylaxis
    b. Bleaching therapy on mandibular arch
    c. Composite on maxillary left incisor
    d. Recall at 6 months
22. Bleaching Ms. O'Bryan's TCN-stained teeth with 10% carbamide peroxide resulted in which of the following outcomes?
    a. Highly sensitive teeth
    b. Noticeable results with long-term bleaching
    c. Excellent short-term whitening results
    d. No whitening effect

23. Given her lack of personal time and desire for whiter teeth, which of the following tooth-whitening systems would you recommend for Ms. Randall?
    a. Tray bleaching
    b. OTC whitening strips
    c. Whitening dentifrice
    d. Laser whitening

WHERE do I go for more information or support?

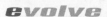

For suggested web sites and agencies, additional readings and resources, and more chapter-specific information, please consult your Evolve Student Resources. Because of the ever-changing nature of the Internet, please keep in mind that web sites listed and their content may change.

 CD-ROM

Reference files: As you work through the CD-ROM exercises, you should be able to print reference files and add them to your class materials. No specific reference files apply to this chapter.

HOW can I keep track of my progress toward competence?

As an ongoing picture of progress, record and monitor clinical experiences relating to Chapter 36 content in your Portfolio.

Self-Reflection

On a regular basis, review these experiences (with a faculty member). Identify strengths, weaknesses (not just numbers), and changes that you would incorporate into your clinical care plan now that you have had these experiences.

37 Orthodontics

WHY do I need to know about Orthodontics?

Dental hygienists have a vital role to play in the diverse and dynamic field of orthodontics, whether they are employed in a general practice environment or in an orthodontic office. Patients often ask dental hygienists questions regarding orthodontic treatment and options. This chapter provides an overview of orthodontic treatments available to consumers.

WHAT will I be able to do with this knowledge?

1. Relate the history and biology of the specialty of orthodontics to dental professionals.
2. Classify malocclusion according to Angle's system.
3. Be aware of the dental hygienist's role in the patient selection and referral for orthodontic treatment.
4. Identify normal ranges of dental development, and recognize deviations from this range.
5. Discuss the three dimensions of the facial structure, and recognize normal and abnormal skeletal structure.
6. Recognize the role of different specialties in interdisciplinary orthodontic treatment.
7. Discuss third molar considerations for postorthodontic recommendations.
8. Instruct orthodontic patients in proper oral hygiene management.
9. Demonstrate your knowledge of orthodontic terms by using them in written and verbal communication.
10. Recognize basic types of treatment components, including those for space management, detrimental oral habits, orthopedic development problems, and orthodontic correction.
11. Recognize general retention devices and guidelines.

HOW do I prepare myself to transfer this knowledge to patient care?

 Go to Chapter 37 content on your CD-ROM or search for "Orthodontics."

CD Exercises

- *37-1: Angle's Classification:* Identify Angle's classification.
- *37-2: Common Orthodontic Appliances Used in Both One-Phase and Two-Phase Treatment:* Identify orthodontic appliances.

Textbook

Review Case Study 37-1, Adult Orthodontics, and the case applications.

For important concepts and application of knowledge, review tables, figures, and boxed sections. The following may be especially helpful for clinical transfer and may be used as a clinical resource:

- Figure 37-1: Pretreatment cephalometric radiograph of patient.
- Figure 37-2: Facial profiles reflecting Class I, II, and III jaw relationships.
- Figure 37-3: Clinical photograph of protrusive maxillary incisors.
- Figure 37-4: Clinical images of a maxillary diastema and low attached frenum before treatment (A); and after orthodontic space closure and frenectomy (B).
- Figure 37-5: Clinical images of a deep bite into palatal gingival.
- Figures 37-6 and 37-7: Histological image of a premolar being moved and compressed periodontal ligament.
- Figure 37-8: Representation of various tooth numbering systems commonly used today.
- Figure 37-9: Facial outline of a patient with Class II malocclusion, before and after treatment.
- Figures 37-10 through 37-24 and 27-38 through 37-31: Various orthodontic fixed and removable appliances.
- Figures 37-25 through 37-27: Clinical images of debonding and removing orthodontic appliances.

HOW do I perform these skills?

evolve

A printable version of this checklist is available on your Evolve Student Resources.

To perform the orthodontic six-point quick check system, I will:

- ☐ Begin by examining *each arch separately* and evaluating these categories:
    1. Arch width (molar-to-molar transpalatal width of 36 mm is average)
    2. Excessive spacing or crowding present
    3. Missing or ankylosed teeth
- ☐ Then note the relationship between the upper and lower teeth in occlusion. Evaluate the following:
    4. Angle's classification
    5. The amount of overbite and overjet present
    6. Any open-bite or cross-bite present

HOW can I more effectively use this knowledge?

Critical Thinking Activities

Use the following worksheet provided to complete activity #1.

1. Perform the orthodontic six-point quick check system on yourself, on a patient in early mixed dentition, and on an adolescent patient. Note Angle's classification for each patient. What are the orthodontic areas of concern noted? Would anyone in the group be a candidate for an orthodontic referral, and why? If anyone in the group is an orthodontic candidate, then what mode of treatment do you think would best treat the orthodontic problem?

2. Visit an orthodontic office to observe patient care. List the duties or positions the dental hygienist would be qualified to perform. If the orthodontist currently employs a hygienist, then interview the hygienist to determine what led him or her to this career choice.

Worksheet #1

Use this form to complete Critical Thinking Activity #1.

	Yourself	Early Mixed Dentition Patient	Adolescent Patient
Six-point quick check system			
Angle's classification			
Orthodontic areas of concern			
Is the patient a candidate for an orthodontic referral? Why?			
What mode of treatment do you think would best treat the orthodontic problem?			

DO I have all the answers?

Review Questions

Check your answers against the Answer Key at the back of this Study Guide to assess what you have learned.

1. At what age does the American Association of Orthodontists recommend that the patient be seen for an initial screening?
   a. 6 to 12 months
   b. Whenever the need arises
   c. 7 years of age
   d. 12 years of age
2. Which one of the following options is a valid reason for choosing a two-phase treatment plan for an adolescent?
   a. Severe crowding
   b. Large anteroposterior discrepancy between the upper and lower jaws
   c. Narrow maxilla, resulting in a cross-bite
   d. Active thumb sucking
   e. All of the above
3. All of the following modes of treatment can be used on an adult orthodontic patient, *except* one. Which one is the *exception?*
   a. Rapid maxillary expansion
   b. Facial mask therapy
   c. Quad helix
   d. Functional orthopedic appliances
   e. Both *b* and *d*
   f. Both *c* and *d*
4. All of the following modes of treatment can be used on a patient in mixed dentition *except* one. Which one is the *exception?*
   a. Quad helix
   b. Orthognathic surgery
   c. Lip bumper
   d. Brackets
5. All of the following should be performed on an orthodontic patient with fixed appliances *except* one. Which one is the *exception?*
   a. Scaling and polishing
   b. Oral hygiene instruction
   c. Tooth bleaching
   d. Topical fluoride application
6. Maxillary midline diastema occurs commonly in which one of the following racial groups?
   a. White
   b. Asian
   c. Black
   d. Hispanic
7. Which one of the following diagnostic aids is *not* a necessary part of preorthodontic records?
   a. Panorex
   b. Cephalometric radiograph
   c. Intraoral photographs
   d. None of the above

8. Severe root resorption is a consequence that is *most likely* caused by which one of the following?
   a. Hereditary factors
   b. Excessive orthodontic force
   c. Root apices contacting cortical bone
   d. Increased length of treatment
9. What average percentage of children receives some type of orthodontic care based on data from the National Health and Nutritional Examination Survey (NHANES III) study?
   a. 5
   b. 75
   c. 30
   d. 50
10. Which of the following factors is *not* part of Angle's classification of malocclusion?
    a. Vertical relationship of teeth
    b. Skeletal relationship of the jaws
    c. Line of occlusion
    d. Both *a* and *b*

WHERE do I go for more information or support?

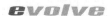

For suggested web sites and agencies, additional readings and resources, and more chapter-specific information, please consult your Evolve Student Resources. Because of the ever-changing nature of the Internet, please keep in mind that web sites listed and their content may change.

CD-ROM

Reference files: As you work through the CD-ROM exercises, you should be able to print reference files and add them to your class materials. No specific reference files apply to this chapter.

HOW can I keep track of my progress toward competence?

As an ongoing picture of progress, record and monitor clinical experiences relating to Chapter 37 content in your Portfolio.

Self-Reflection

On a regular basis, review these experiences (with a faculty member). Identify strengths, weaknesses (not just numbers), and changes that you would incorporate into your clinical care plan now that you have had these experiences.

38 Oral Malodor Diagnosis and Management

WHY do I need to know about Oral Malodor Diagnosis and Management?

Oral malodor is a common condition that will be encountered daily in clinical practice. The dental hygienist must be able to integrate oral malodor management strategies throughout the preventive and therapeutic appointment. In addition to the obvious unpleasantness associated with oral malodor, the connection between oral malodor and periodontal disease may also provide key motivational opportunities to achieve optimal oral health.

WHAT will I be able to do with this knowledge?

1. Differentiate among the etiologies associated with malodor.
2. Identify the intraoral niches involved in the production of oral malodor.
3. Explain the relationship between oral malodor and periodontal disease.
4. Establish clinical management protocols for oral malodor.
5. Discriminate among various mechanical and chemotherapeutic methods for oral malodor treatment and prevention.
6. Identify methods to discuss professionally the topic of oral malodor with patients.

HOW do I prepare myself to transfer this knowledge to patient care?

 Go to Chapter 38 content on your CD-ROM or search for "Malodor."

CD Exercises

- *38-1: Malodor Etiology:* Match the type of odor with the most likely cause.
- *38-2: Malodor Etiology:* Assess the following patients for risk of malodor based on their history: Ann Cronin, George Burkett, Subra Mani, and Adolfo Santana.

Textbook

Review Case Study 38-1, Oral Malodor Management, and the case applications.

For important concepts and application of knowledge, tables, figures, and boxed sections listed here may be especially helpful for clinical transfer and may be used as a clinical reference:

- Box 38–1: Periodontal Infection and Oral Malodor
- Box 38-2: Organoleptic Intensity Scale
- Box 38-4: Tongue Deplaquing Procedure
- Box 38-5: Active Agents for Neutralizing Volatile Sulfur Compounds and Controlling Gram-Negative Oral Flora
- Box 38-6: Discussing Oral Malodor During the Dental Hygiene Experience
- Box 38-7: Oral Hygiene Recommendations for Reduction of Oral Malodor
- Figure 38-3 shows deplaquing of the tongue at the conclusion of the appointment.
- Figures 38-9 and 38-10 show tongue deplaquing.

HOW do I perform these skills?

evolve

A printable version of this checklist is available on your Evolve Student Resources.
To utilize successfully the suggested process of care that includes integration of oral malodor assessment and treatment with traditional dental hygiene treatment protocols, I will:

Assessment Phase

- ☐ Review medical history.
  - ☐ Ask questions regarding family history of systemic illnesses, xerostomia, or medications that contribute to oral malodor.
- ☐ Review current oral hygiene routine.
  - ☐ Assess *real* time and tools used, as well as technique.
- ☐ Determine current usage and frequency of usage of oral malodor–related products.
  - ☐ Toothpaste: Specific brand and times per day
  - ☐ Mouthrinse: Specific brand, times per day, and amount of time rinsing
  - ☐ Breath Mints: Specific brand and times per day
  - ☐ Chewing Gum: Specific brand and times per day
  - ☐ Other: Tongue gels, breath sprays, etc.
- ☐ Perform oral cancer screening.
  - ☐ Note that oral lesions can emit odor.

□ Perform comprehensive periodontal examination.
  □ Pocket depths of 4 mm or greater are more likely to produce volatile sulfur compounds (VSCs).
□ Note the condition of the surface of the tongue.
  □ Tongue coating in periodontal patients is four to six times greater.
□ Identify restorations, crown, or bridges that need replacing.
  □ These plaque biofilm–retentive areas can produce oral malodor.
□ Note the presence of oral lesions and tonsilloliths.
  □ Tonsil stones have a malodor component.

Clinical Protocol

□ Use preprocedural and postprocedural antibacterial mouthrinse to neutralize VSCs.
□ Eliminate or reduce plaque biofilm and calculus.
  □ Nonperiodontal
  □ Full-mouth debridement (FMD) protocol for periodontal cases
  □ Instrumentation as indicated
  □ Subgingival irrigation to neutralize VSC via automated scalers or other irrigation device
  □ Removing remaining plaque biofilm from interproximal regions
  □ Performing selective polishing as indicated
  □ Performing tongue deplaquing procedure using tongue scraper and antibacterial or VSC neutralizing agent
□ Evaluate for additional preventive care.
  □ Instruct patient on daily care for fresh breath maintenance and make product recommendations.
  □ Reappoint as indicated and evaluate fresh breath success.

Tongue Deplaquing Procedure

□ With the patient observing the procedure, have him or her extend the tongue and place an antibacterial agent to the surface of the tongue.
□ Apply light pressure and place the tongue-cleaning device as far posterior on the surface of the tongue as possible.
□ Gently move the cleaning device forward, and remove the tongue coating or debris via suction or 2 × 2 gauze square. Repeat as needed.
□ Take the opportunity to explain that this process will help reduce oral malodor when implemented on a daily basis.

HOW can I more effectively use this knowledge?

Critical Thinking Activities

1. Survey 10 colleagues and have them complete the following exercise: Thoroughly brush the surface of the tongue. After this exercise, ask them to use a tongue-cleaning device. Solicit comments from the colleagues about the two cleaning methods. List the comments for each method. Consider how you could incorporate these comments into patient education.

2. Visit a local drug store and inventory products targeting oral malodor other than toothpastes, toothbrushes, flosses, and mouthrinses. Determine sugar content, active ingredients, and directions for use. Consider the marketplace and consumer interest and how these factors may assist in facilitating optimal oral health.

3. Use the Internet and search for the terms *bad breath* and *halitosis*. Note the number of web resources dedicated to this condition, and contemplate your role in fresh-breath assurance.

DO I have all the answers?

Review Questions

Check your answers against the Answer Key at the back of this Study Guide to assess what you have learned.

1. Approximately 80% of oral malodor is related to which one of the following?
   a. Halitosis
   b. Oral environment
   c. Systemic-based malodor
   d. Food, medications, tobacco

2. Tongue scraping and deplaquing will reduce VSCs by 75% and is more effective than tongue brushing.
   a. The first part of the statement is true; the second part is false.
   b. Both parts of the statement are true.
   c. The first part of the statement is false; the second part is true.
   d. Both parts of the statement are false.

3. Which one of the following options is the odor-causing component to bad breath?
   a. Gram-negative anaerobic bacteria
   b. Gram-positive bacteria
   c. VSCs
   d. Metabolized protein

4. Gram-negative anaerobic bacteria are associated with which one of the following oral infections?
   a. Dental caries
   b. Gingivitis
   c. Periodontal disease
   d. All of the above

5. Which of the following VSCs is associated with periodontal disease?
   a. Hydrogen sulfide
   b. Methyl mercaptan
   c. Dimethyl sulfide
   d. Dimethyl disulfide

6. Which one of the following VSCs is associated with patients who do not have periodontal disease?
   a. Hydrogen sulfide
   b. Methyl mercaptan
   c. Dimethyl sulfide
   d. Dimethyl disulfide

7. VSCs' role in the progression of periodontal disease includes which one of the following items?
   a. Increase in permeability of oral mucosa and penetration of endotoxin
   b. Suppression of DNA synthesis

c. Interference with collagen and protein synthesis
d. All of the above
e. None of the above

8. Which one of the following options best describes zinc's main mechanism of action?
   a. Kills gram-negative bacteria
   b. Kills gram-positive bacteria
   c. Neutralizes VSCs
   d. Decreases cell permeability

9. Bacteria associated with bad breath can be found in all of the following anatomical components *except* one. Which one is the *exception?*
   a. Buccal mucosa
   b. Subgingivally
   c. Posterior dorsum of the tongue
   d. Tonsils

10. Oral malodor management requires all of the following items *except* one. Which one is the *exception?*
    a. Decreasing salivary flow
    b. Eliminating gram-negative bacteria
    c. Neutralizing VSCs
    d. Daily tongue deplaquing

For suggested web sites and agencies, additional readings and resources, and more chapter-specific information, please consult your Evolve Student Resources. Because of the ever-changing nature of the Internet, please keep in mind that web sites listed and their content may change.

CD-ROM

Reference files: As you work through the CD-ROM exercises, you should be able to print reference files and add them to your class materials. No specific reference files apply to this chapter.

HOW can I keep track of my progress toward competence?

As an ongoing picture of progress, record and monitor clinical experiences relating to Chapter 38 content in your Portfolio.

Self-Reflection

On a regular basis, review these experiences (with a faculty member). Identify strengths, weaknesses (not just numbers), and changes that you would incorporate into your clinical care plan now that you have had these experiences.

39 Emergency Management of Dental Trauma

WHY do I need to know about Emergency Management of Dental Trauma?

Dental hygienists have the knowledge and skill to recognize dental and nondental conditions that place a child or adult at risk for oral trauma. Dental hygienists can help expand the scope of trauma prevention and, through recognition of trauma, can prevent future occurrences to a victim.

WHAT will I be able to do with this knowledge?

1. Discuss the epidemiologic and etiologic factors of dental trauma.
2. Perform appropriate physical and oral assessments of traumatized dental patients.
3. Describe appropriate protocols for emergency management or referral of patients with dental injuries.
4. Outline proper documentation for traumatized dental patients.
5. Understand strategies for the prevention of orofacial trauma, with particular emphasis on child abuse and sports-related dental injuries.

HOW do I prepare myself to transfer this knowledge to patient care?

 Go to Chapter 39 content on your CD-ROM or search for "Dental Trauma."

CD Exercises

- *39-1: Emergency Management of Dental Trauma:* Determine whether statements presented reflect incidence or prevalence.
- *39-2: Developmental Etiology:* Select facial profiles most prone to injury.
- *39-3 to 39-4: Developmental Etiology:* Identify oral risk for Terrence Zellar based on patient records.
- *39-5 to 39-6: Sports Related Injury—Adolfo Santana:* Select the appropriate sports-related prevention mechanism, based on patient records.
- *39-7 to 39-8: Risk Assessment—Eva Bjork:* Select appropriate trauma evaluation methods.
- *39-9: Emergency Management of Dental Trauma:* Select the appropriate treatment of avulsion of primary tooth.
- *39-10: Child Abuse and Neglect:* Place in chronologic order a timeline of child protection mandates.

Textbook

Review Case Study 39-1, Sports-Related Dental Trauma, and the case applications.

For important concepts and application of knowledge, tables and boxed sections listed here may be especially helpful for clinical transfer and may be used as a clinical resource:

- Table 39-1: Procedure Codes Associated with Mouth Trauma
- Box 39-1: Questions to Ask or Consider While Examining a Suspected Abuse Victim

HOW do I perform these skills?

evolve

A printable version of this checklist is available on your Evolve Student Resources.

Questions I will ask or consider while examining a suspected abuse victim:

- ☐ How did the injury occur?
- ☐ When did it occur?
- ☐ Has the child had similar injuries on several occasions?
- ☐ Does the child have a repeated history of hospitalizations, often at different hospitals?
- ☐ Has the parent or guardian delayed seeking treatment?
- ☐ Does the child act inappropriately to the invasion of personal space by the dental professional?
- ☐ Is the parent or guardian hostile or blaming or claiming that the child's behavior is different?
- ☐ Does a young child accuse someone?
- ☐ Does an older child seem reluctant or fearful to say anything when asked what or how the injury occurred?
- ☐ Is the child dirty or inappropriately dressed for the season?
- ☐ Does evidence exist of old injuries (e.g., marks, bruising at various stages of healing)?
- ☐ Does any evidence exist of burns?
- ☐ Does any evidence exist of injury to the back of the legs, orbital area, mouth, ears, or face in general; torn frenal attachments; palatal petechia; and/or fractured or avulsed teeth?

HOW can I more effectively use this knowledge?

Critical Thinking Activities

1. Fabricate a type II *boil-and-bite* mouthguard. Evaluate the finished mouthguard for protective qualities.
2. Volunteer to participate in a local *mouthguard day*. Observe the ages of persons who are interested in information. In which sporting activities are they involved?
3. Participate in a local Special Olympics Special Smiles program event.
4. Review course availability on domestic violence and child abuse. Prepare a handout for students and faculty to encourage them to attend a class.
5. Interview an abuse counselor. Determine his or her experiences with trauma to the head and neck region of abuse victims, differentiating among men, women, children, and older adults.
6. Obtain a child abuse and neglect report from your appropriate local authority.
7. Review your state's dental practice act to determine your legal obligations in reporting suspected child abuse and neglect.

DO I have all the answers?

Review Questions

Check your answers against the Answer Key at the back of this Study Guide to assess what you have learned.
Questions 2 through 5 refer to Case Study 39-1.

1. Dental hygienists play a key role in primary care prevention in the dental office and through community service projects. Which one of the following activities should be included in a total dental prevention program?
   a. Prevention of dental caries
   b. Prevention of periodontal diseases
   c. Prevention of traumatic dental injuries
   d. Prevention of child abuse and neglect
   e. All of the above
2. When Ms. Washington's mother contacts your trauma-ready dental office, which one of the following sets of instructions should she be given to enhance the prognosis for her daughter's avulsed permanent incisor?
   a. Reinsert the avulsed tooth into the socket, and bring Ms. Washington to the dental office immediately.
   b. Place the tooth in milk, and bring Ms. Washington and her avulsed tooth to the dental office within the next 2 days.
   c. Control the bleeding, place the avulsed tooth in a dry paper towel, and bring Ms. Washington and her avulsed tooth to the dental office immediately.
   d. Control the bleeding, and bring Ms. Washington to the dental office within the next 2 days.

3. When Ms. Washington arrives at the dental office, which one of the following diagnostic procedures should *not* be performed in her case of an avulsed permanent incisor?
   a. Updated health history
   b. Clinical examination
   c. Percussion of avulsed tooth
   d. Periapical radiograph
4. After the dentist has repositioned and splinted the avulsed tooth in place, which one of the following oral self-care instructions should the dental hygienist give to Ms. Washington and her mother?
   a. Avoid brushing and flossing the traumatized tooth and soft tissue, but continue to brush and floss the remainder of the teeth.
   b. Vigorously brush and floss the traumatized tooth and soft tissue with a hard toothbrush, and use an interproximal dental stimulator.
   c. Avoid brushing and flossing for the 2 weeks that the splint is in place.
   d. Gently brush and floss the traumatized tooth and soft tissue with a soft toothbrush, and use an intraoral rinse such as warm salt water or chlorhexidine. Maintain standard oral self-care for the remainder of the teeth.
5. Which one of the following recommendations should be made to Ms. Washington and her mother in terms of Ms. Washington's future participation in athletic activities?
   a. Stop playing basketball.
   b. Play basketball less vigorously.
   c. Use a properly fitted mouthguard when playing basketball.
   d. Switch to a different sport, such as field hockey.

WHERE do I go for more information or support?

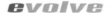

For suggested web sites and agencies, additional readings and resources, and more chapter-specific information, please consult your Evolve Student Resources. Because of the ever-changing nature of the Internet, please keep in mind that web sites listed and their content may change.

 CD-ROM

Reference files: As you work through the CD-ROM exercises, you should be able to print reference files and add them to your class materials. No specific reference files apply to this chapter.

HOW can I keep track of my progress toward competence?

As an ongoing picture of progress, record and monitor clinical experiences relating to Chapter 39 content in your Portfolio:

When seeing a patient who may have a history of dental trauma, ask him or her how the situation was managed, and evaluate the long-term effects of this management strategy.

Keep track of any dental trauma cases that may be seen in clinic, and evaluate what type of actions were taken to manage the situation.

Keep track of recommendations and instructions given to parents and children regarding trauma management, bite guard fabrication, or other measures.

Develop a dialog and course of action that you can use when abuse or neglect is suspected.

Self-Reflection

On a regular basis, review these experiences (with a faculty member). Identify strengths, weaknesses (not just numbers), and changes that you would incorporate into your clinical care plan now that you have had these experiences.

40 Anxiety Control

WHY do I need to know about Anxiety Control?

The dental hygienist is in a key position to affect the oral health of all patients positively by helping them cope with their anxieties regarding dental treatment.

WHAT will I be able to do with this knowledge?

1. Differentiate the terms *phobia, fear,* and *anxiety.*
2. Analyze patient responses to questions in the dental history designed to detect anxiety about treatment.
3. Identify the origin of a patient's anxiety through questioning during the initial assessment phase of treatment.
4. Identify and evaluate fear-provoking situations with a patient.
5. Recognize the signs and behaviors that indicate dental anxiety.
6. Evaluate the reliability of tools used to assess dental anxiety.
7. Understand nonpharmacologic strategies that can help patients of all ages develop coping skills for handling their anxiety.
8. Formulate a personalized treatment plan for an anxious patient based on his or her particular circumstances, goals, and level and type of anxiety.

HOW do I prepare myself to transfer this knowledge to patient care?

 Go to Chapter 40 content on your CD-ROM or search for "Anxiety Control."

CD Exercises

- *40-1: Behavioral Management of Anxiety:* Through video demonstration, identify psychologic management techniques.
- *40-2 and 40-3: Behavioral Management of Anxiety— Eva Bjork:* Select anxiety management techniques based on patient needs for Eva Bjork.
- *40-4: Behavioral Management of Anxiety—Elena Guri:* Select anxiety management techniques based on patient needs for Elena Guri.

Textbook

Review Case Study 40-1, Identification and Management of Dental Anxiety, and the case applications.

For important concepts and application of knowledge, boxes and figures listed here may be especially helpful for clinical transfer and may be used as a clinical resource:
- Box 40-1: Anxious Behaviors in the Reception Area
- Box 40-2: Sample Dental History Questions Designed to Identify Anxiety
- Box 40-3: Sample Initial Interview Questions Related to Dental Anxiety
- Box 40-4: Guided Relaxation
- Box 40-5: Systematic Desensitization Hierarchy for Tooth Probing
- Figure 40-1: Negative cyclical pattern of dental anxiety.
- Figure 40-2: Dental anxiety scale—revised (DAS-R).

HOW can I more effectively use this knowledge?

Critical Thinking Activities

Use the following worksheet to complete activity #7.
1. Invite a guest speaker to discuss and demonstrate hypnosis.
2. Develop video recordings for different age groups to be used for modeling purposes.
3. Use distraction methods by encouraging patients to bring in headsets and audio recordings.
4. Produce a relaxation audio recording for use with clinic patients.
5. Use other relaxation techniques with clinic patients.
6. Practice relaxation techniques to help yourself manage the stress in your life.
7. Through discussion, attempt to identify the origin of a patient's anxiety. Review patients on the CD-ROM, and enter your answers on Worksheet #1.
8. Create a stimulus hierarchy for nonsurgical periodontal therapy.
9. With a fellow student, role-play the treatment of an anxious patient. Focus on interpersonal characteristics, communication, and patient control enhancement.
10. Using the DAS-R, identify the number of anxious patients treated in a given month.

Worksheet #1

Use this form to complete Critical Thinking Activity #7. Determine which of the patients on the CD-ROM suffer from anxiety and the best treatment approach for a dental examination procedure.

Patient Name	Anxiety Identification	Care Planning Modifications	Behavioral Management Techniques

DO I have all the answers?

Review Questions

Check your answers against the Answer Key at the back of this Study Guide to assess what you have learned. Questions 1 and 2 refer to Case Study 40-1.

1. Which one of the following behaviors suggests that Ms. Uri is anxious about oral care?
   a. Previous cancellation
   b. Aloofness
   c. Lack of preventive care
   d. Poor oral health
   e. All of the above
2. Which one of the following interventions should be provided first for Ms. Uri?
   a. Guided use of a muscle relaxation technique
   b. An explanation of the procedure
   c. Administration of an anxiety questionnaire
   d. Referral to a mental health professional
3. Which one of the following strategies would probably be most successful for anxious 3- to 5-year-old children?
   a. Modeling
   b. Detailed explanations
   c. Coaxing
   d. Paced breathing
4. Which one of the following techniques requires creating a hierarchy of fear-producing situations?
   a. Hypnosis
   b. Systematic desensitization
   c. Biofeedback
   d. Progressive muscle relaxation
5. Which one of the following factors has the greatest influence on the patient's perception of the oral care experience?
   a. Achievement of complete relaxation
   b. Detailed information about the proposed treatment
   c. Interpersonal relationship between the patient and the care provider
   d. Quality care delivered in an efficient manner

WHERE do I go for more information or support?

evolve

For suggested web sites and agencies, additional readings and resources, and more chapter-specific information, please consult your Evolve Student Resources. Because of the ever-changing nature of the Internet, please keep in mind that web sites listed and their content may change.

CD-ROM

Reference files: As you work through the CD-ROM exercises, you should be able to print reference files and add them to your class materials. No specific reference files apply to this chapter.

HOW can I keep track of my progress toward competence?

As an ongoing picture of progress, record and monitor clinical experiences relating to Chapter 40 content in your Portfolio:

Review anxiety prevention strategies that you have used on patients in clinic to help determine which works best in various situations.

- Observe faculty and classmates when dealing with anxious patients to help understand strategies and develop protocols that will work for you.
- Record situations that you have encountered with anxious patients so that you can look back on these situations and review them at a later date to determine effectiveness of outcomes.

Self-Reflection

On a regular basis, review these experiences (with a faculty member). Identify strengths, weaknesses (not just numbers), and changes that you would incorporate into your clinical care plan now that you have had these experiences.

41 Local Anesthetics

WHY do I need to know about Local Anesthetics?

Local anesthetics are used in dentistry primarily to manage pain experienced by the patient during treatment procedures. The dental hygienist is responsible for monitoring the status of the patient who has received a local anesthetic agent and is receiving treatment from the hygienist. Where allowed by state law, dental hygienists deliver local anesthetics during patient care, as well as anesthetize a patient in preparation for restorative therapy or surgery as directed by a dentist.

WHAT will I be able to do with this knowledge?

1. Describe the uses of local anesthetics in the practice of dental hygiene.
2. Name the first local anesthetic, and explain why it is no longer the drug of choice.
3. Describe the physiologic mechanism of nerve conduction.
4. Explain how local anesthetics block nerve conduction.
5. Describe the chemical classes of local anesthetics.
6. Discuss the effect pH has on local anesthetics.
7. Describe the pharmacokinetics of local anesthetics.
8. Identify the systemic actions of local anesthetics.
9. Discuss the purpose of adding a vasoconstrictor to a local anesthetic solution.
10. Describe the clinical action of specific local anesthetics.
11. Select the correct armamentarium for individual injections.
12. Describe the basic steps involved in the delivery of a local anesthetic injection.
13. Understand the general principles of technique and safety.
14. Recognize the anatomical landmarks associated with the common local anesthetic injections.
15. Describe all major maxillary and mandibular injection techniques used in dental hygiene practice.
16. Discuss the potential local and systemic complications related to the delivery of local anesthetic agents.

HOW do I prepare myself to transfer this knowledge to patient care?

 Go to Chapter 41 content on your CD-ROM or search for "Anesthetic."

CD Exercises

- *41-1: Overview of Commonly Used Local Anesthetic Agents:* Identify types of anesthetics and their delivery vehicles.
- *41-2: Administration of Local and Topical Anesthetic Agents—Ann Cronin:* Select type of topical and injectable agent based on patient record of Ann Cronin.
- *41-3: Administration of Local and Topical Anesthetic Agents:* Select the correct nerve block.
- *41-4: Administration of Local and Topical Anesthetic Agents:* Review selection of needle and site. Student is asked to select appropriate needle and site for use.
- *41-5: Administration of Local and Topical Anesthetic Agents—Ann Cronin:* Select method of injection based on patient needs for Ann Cronin.
- *41-6: Documentation of Local Anesthetic Agents— George Burkett:* Make correct chart notation based on scenario for George Burkett.

Textbook

Review Case Study 41-1, Anesthesia Considerations, and the case applications.

Tables and boxed material listed here may be especially helpful for clinical transfer and may be used as a clinical resource:

- Distinct Care Modifications Boxes
- Box 41-1: Contents of a Typical Local Anesthetic Cartridge
- Box 41-2: American Dental Association Standards for Syringes
- Box 41-3: Sample Chart Documentation for Local Anesthetics
- Table 41-1 lists the local anesthetic drugs currently available in dental cartridges.
- Tables 41-2 and 41-3 provide a summary of the key elements of each injection.

HOW do I perform these skills?

evolve

A printable version of this checklist is available on your Evolve Student Resources.

To administer an injectable and topical anesthetic correctly, I will:

Injection

- □ Review health history.
- □ Obtain informed consent for patient treatment.
- □ Identify area to be anesthetized.
- □ Select appropriate needle gauge and length.
- □ Select proper anesthetic based on health history.
- □ Properly load cartridge into syringe.
- □ Ensure that the plunger on an aspirating syringe engages the rubber stopper with a harpoon or hook and makes it possible to pull back on the stopper, creating negative pressure inside the cartridge.
- □ Attach needle.
- □ Conduct an aspiration test.
- □ Apply topical anesthetic as needed.
- □ Wait appropriate length of time to allow for topical effect.
- □ Administer the local anesthetic.
- □ Use scoop technique to recap needle.
- □ Observe patient for adverse reaction.
- □ Set patient expectations (outcomes).
- □ Document findings and procedure or procedures in chart.

Topical Application

- □ Review health history.
- □ Select appropriate topical anesthetic.
- □ Identify area to be anesthetized.
- □ Dry area to be anesthetized.
- □ Apply topical anesthetic with cotton-tipped applicator.
- □ If before the injection, wait appropriate length of time to allow for topical effect.
- □ Document findings and procedure in chart.

HOW can I more effectively use this knowledge?

Critical Thinking Activities

Use the following worksheet to complete activity #2.

1. Select an anesthetic and review the literature for the following:
   a. Allergic reactions
   b. Preservatives and reactions
   c. Duration of anesthesia
   d. Doses available
   e. Other properties
2. Select two of the reviews from Critical Thinking Activity #1, and complete Worksheet #1.
3. Apply a topical anesthetic to a cotton-tipped applicator. Place it on the floor of a fellow student's mouth for 10 seconds (providing no medical contraindications exist), and then remove it. Determine the amount of time required for the anesthetic effect to subside.
4. Review the dental records of three patients who were given a local anesthetic for dental procedures. Record the information the same way the dosage notations were made in the record.

Worksheet #1

After completing Critical Thinking Activity #2, use this form to review one dentifrice and one additional type of desensitizing therapy.

OVERVIEW

Article title _____

Author(s) _____

Publication title _____

Date, volume, issue, page _____

Stated purpose of the study _____

What was being evaluated? _____

METHODOLOGY

Study Design

Was the study design clearly described and appropriate for the investigation? _____

_____

Was the study design double blind? _____

Was the study design single blind? _____

Was the length of investigation sufficient to study the subject? _____

Was interexaminer and intraexaminer reliability stated? _____

Subjects

Was the sample size large enough? _____

Composition of the sample population: Was it appropriate to the therapy used? _____

How many subjects dropped out of the study (through attrition)? _____

Did the researchers attempt to balance the groups? _____

Continued

Worksheet #1—cont'd

After completing Critical Thinking Activity #2, use this form to review one dentifrice and one additional type of desensitizing therapy.

OVERVIEW

Article title _____

Author(s) _____

Publication title _____

Date, volume, issue, page _____

Stated purpose of the study _____

What was being evaluated? _____

METHODOLOGY

Study Design

Was the study design clearly described and appropriate for the investigation? _____

_____

Was the study design double blind? _____

Was the study design single blind? _____

Was the length of investigation sufficient to study the subject? _____

Was interexaminer and intraexaminer reliability stated? _____

Subjects

Was the sample size large enough? _____

Composition of the sample population: Was it appropriate to the therapy used? _____

How many subjects dropped out of the study (through attrition)? _____

Did the researchers attempt to balance the groups? _____

210

DO I have all the answers?

Review Questions

Check your answers against the Answer Key at the back of this Study Guide to assess what you have learned.

1. In comparing a 25-gauge needle with a 30-gauge needle, the 25-gauge needle:
    1. Provides for better aspiration
    2. Breaks more easily
    3. Is less comfortable than the 30-gauge needle
    4. Has a smaller diameter
    5. Can be used in highly vascular areas
    a. *2, 4,* and *5*
    b. *2* and *4*
    c. *1, 3,* and *5*
    d. *1* and *5*

2. What mechanism is responsible for the repolarization of a nerve after it has fired off an impulse?
    a. Nodes of Ranvier
    b. Sodium pump
    c. Specific receptor sites
    d. Bradykinin release
    e. Membrane expansion

3. Anesthetic injected into infected tissue is less effective because:
    a. The infection breaks down the anesthetic.
    b. None of the anesthetic diffuses through the nerve membrane.
    c. The increased blood flow immediately carries all of the anesthetic away.
    d. Fewer base molecules of anesthetic are available to diffuse through the nerve membrane.

4. The causes of trismus might include which one of the following factors?
    a. Excessive volumes of local anesthetics injected into a restricted area
    b. Alcohol diffused into the anesthetic cartridge
    c. Low-grade infection caused by contaminated needles
    d. Hematoma
    e. All of the above

WHERE do I go for more information or support?

 evolve

For suggested web sites and agencies, additional readings and resources, and more chapter-specific information, please consult your Evolve Student Resources. Because of the ever-changing nature of the Internet, please keep in mind that web sites listed and their content may change.

CD-ROM

Reference files: As you work through the CD-ROM exercises, you should be able to print reference files and add them to your class materials. No specific reference files apply to this chapter.

HOW can I keep track of my progress toward competence?

As an ongoing picture of progress, record and monitor clinical experiences relating to Chapter 41 content in your Portfolio.

Self-Reflection

On a regular basis, review these experiences (with a faculty member). Identify strengths, weaknesses (not just numbers), and changes that you would incorporate into your clinical care plan now that you have had these experiences.

42 Nitrous Oxide and Oxygen Sedation

WHY do I need to know about Nitrous Oxide and Oxygen Sedation?

The dental hygienist will often encounter patients who are anxious about dental treatment. To manage both pain and anxiety effectively, a dental hygienist must have an understanding of the available options. Nitrous oxide (N_2O) and oxygen (O_2) sedation is a safe and effective method proven to be applicable to most patients without any significant side effects. Knowledge of the indications for use, effects, pharmacologic equipment, techniques for administration, and patient responses is critical to the safe use of this form of sedation.

WHAT will I be able to do with this knowledge?

1. Appreciate the history of N_2O use and its association with the dental profession.
2. Identify the effects of N_2O on pain, anxiety, and the body's systems.
3. Understand the properties of N_2O.
4. Explain indications and relative contraindications for the use of N_2O/O_2 sedation.
5. Identify equipment associated with N_2O/O_2 sedation.
6. Describe the appropriate technique for N_2O/O_2 administration.
7. Recognize the signs and symptoms of ideal sedation and oversedation.
8. Recognize appropriate recovery from N_2O/O_2 sedation.
9. Separate the facts from fallacies associated with chronic exposure to N_2O.
10. Describe methods for the detection and assessment of trace levels of N_2O in the dental setting.
11. Describe methods to minimize trace levels of N_2O in the dental setting.

HOW do I prepare myself to transfer this knowledge to patient care?

 Go to Chapter 42 content on your CD-ROM or search for "Nitrous Oxide."

CD Exercises

- *42-1: Relative Contraindications:* List eight contraindications of N_2O/O_2 sedation.
- *42-2: Indications or Relative Contraindications—Seven Patients:* Select the patients who are appropriate for N_2O/O_2 sedation.

- *42-3: Oversedation:* Determine characteristics of oversedation.
- *42-4: Biological Effects and Issues:* Respond to true and false questions regarding N_2O/O_2 sedation.

Textbook

Review Case Study 42-1, Administration of Nitrous Oxide and Oxygen Sedation, and the case applications.

For important concepts and application of knowledge, the table and listed here may be especially helpful for clinical transfer and may be used as a clinical reference:

- Table 42-1: Nitrous Oxide/Oxygen Percentage Chart
- Box 42-1: Documentation after Use of Nitrous Oxide/Oxygen Sedation

HOW do I perform these skills?

evolve

A printable version of this checklist is available on your Evolve Student Resources.

To administer N_2O/O_2 sedation successfully, I will:

- ☐ Review health history for contraindications.
- ☐ Explain the procedure and effect of treatment.
- ☐ Obtain informed consent for treatment.
- ☐ Check all equipment for proper functioning.
- ☐ Select the appropriate size and type of nasal hood for the patient.
- ☐ Secure the hood to the conduction tubing.
- ☐ Administer proper oxygen flow to the unit.
- ☐ Properly titrate nitrous oxide.
- ☐ Adjust levels to proper liter flow per minute.
- ☐ At treatment completion, provide patient with postoperative oxygen.
- ☐ Terminate nitrous oxide flow.
- ☐ Continue the oxygen flow until patient feels completely normal.
- ☐ Document appropriate treatment notes for use of nitrous oxide.
- ☐ Set patient expectations (outcomes).
- ☐ Document findings and procedure in chart.

HOW can I more effectively use this knowledge?

Critical Thinking Activities

1. Investigate the status of nitrous oxide and oxygen (N_2O/O_2) administration by hygienists in your state's dental practice act. Determine the requirements (e.g., number of course hours, supervision levels, fees) for practicing this skill in your state.
2. Debate the pros and cons of using N_2O/O_2 sedation in dental hygiene care.
3. Develop a persuasive paper on the use of N_2O/O_2 sedation in dental hygiene care.
4. Visit dental offices, and identify the type of N_2O/O_2 equipment used.
5. Check with supply houses to determine the cost of various tank sizes of N_2O and O_2.

DO I have all the answers?

Review Questions

Check your answers against the Answer Key at the back of this Study Guide to assess what you have learned. Questions 3 through 6 refer to Case Study 42-1.

1. N_2O pressure in the tank will not show a decrease on the gauge until the _____ phase is nearly gone and primarily _____ remains in the tank.
   a. Liquid; vapor
   b. Gas; liquid
   c. Liquid; water
   d. Gas; vapor
2. Oversedation includes all of the following signs *except* one. Which sign is the *exception?*
   a. Tingling sensation in extremities
   b. Sweating
   c. Dizziness
   d. Inability to keep mouth open
   e. Increased sleepiness
3. Mr. Gruenwald heard that a person with allergies or asthma should not use N_2O/O_2 sedation, and he is concerned because he has some allergies. Your response could be any of the following factors *except* which one?
   a. N_2O is nonirritating to mucosa in the respiratory system.
   b. No documented allergy to N_2O has occurred in more than 150 years.
   c. Occasionally, asthma attacks occur in nervous or anxious people, therefore N_2O/O_2 sedation is beneficial for these patients.
   d. N_2O can initiate an asthmatic attack because it irritates bronchial tissues.
4. During Mr. Gruenwald's care experience with N_2O/O_2 sedation, the dental hygienist can monitor his respiration by which one of the following?
   a. Adjusting the N_2O amount being delivered
   b. Checking the pressure gauges on the equipment
   c. Observing the movement of the reservoir bag
   d. Watching the floating balls in the flowmeter tubes

5. Mr. Gruenwald has had a positive experience with N_2O/O_2 sedation and is ready to be dismissed. He is wondering how long the N_2O stays in his system. You assure him that N_2O is quickly eliminated by which one of the following?
   a. Kidneys
   b. Skin
   c. Lungs
   d. Liver
   e. Urine
6. As you assess Mr. Gruenwald's recovery from N_2O/O_2 sedation, which one of the following would indicate that his recovery may not yet be complete?
   a. You have administered 5 minutes of 100% oxygen postoperatively, and he is feeling normal.
   b. His postoperative vital signs are within close range of his preoperative values.
   c. He says that it seems like his appointment went quickly and that it did not feel like he was at the office very long.
   d. He says he feels groggy and still "out of it."
7. Providing N_2O/O_2 sedation for patients is an important part of your office philosophy. It is also important that the office staff follows an established routine for checking the equipment and making sure all scavenging devices are appropriately working. You follow the guidelines set by the manufacturers and send the flowmeters back to the company for evaluation over which period?
   a. 6 months
   b. 1 year
   c. 2 years
   d. 5 years
8. Scavenging trace gas from the dental office can be accomplished in all the following ways *except* one. Which one is the *exception?*
   a. Adequate suction system that vents to an outside source
   b. Recirculating exhaust ventilation system
   c. Oscillating floor fans directed away from the operator
   d. Regular inspection of equipment for leakage
   e. Use of scavenging mask and nasal hood
9. All of the following are relative contraindications for N_2O/O_2 sedation *except* one. Which one is the *exception?*
   a. Hypersensitive gag reflex
   b. Severely claustrophobic patients
   c. Current upper respiratory infection
   d. First trimester of pregnancy
   e. Alcohol intoxication or drug use

WHERE do I go for more information or support?

evolve

For suggested web sites and agencies, additional readings and resources, and more chapter-specific information, please consult your Evolve Student Resources. Because of the ever-changing nature of the Internet, please keep in mind that web sites listed and their content may change.

 CD-ROM

Reference files: As you work through the CD-ROM exercises, you should be able to print reference files and add them to your class materials. No specific reference files apply to this chapter.

HOW can I keep track of my progress toward competence?

As an ongoing picture of progress, record and monitor clinical experiences relating to Chapter 42 content in your Portfolio:

Keep track of patients who might benefit from nitrous oxide, even though this may not be an available option in the clinic.

Develop a dialog to use with patients that will help them understand the benefits and effects of nitrous oxide, and keep it as a resource or patient education pamphlet.

Self-Reflection

On a regular basis, review these experiences (with a faculty member). Identify strengths, weaknesses (not just numbers), and changes that you would incorporate into your clinical care plan now that you have had these experiences.

43 Saliva and Salivary Dysfunction

WHY do I need to know about Saliva and Salivary Dysfunction?

Saliva is one of the body fluids that provides protection, nutrients, and hydration to the body. The dental hygienist can provide better individualized patient treatment from understanding the functions of saliva and the components that make this fluid unique. Current and future diagnoses of illness are and will continue to be discovered through examination of this fluid.

WHAT will I be able to do with this knowledge?

1. Understand the functions of saliva in maintaining oral health.
2. Describe some of the constituents of saliva and their contribution to the oral cavity.
3. Know the classification of the salivary glands according to their type of secretion.
4. Recognize information in a patient's health history that may be related to salivary gland dysfunction.
5. Identify patients with decreased salivary function by (1) asking specific questions, (2) assessing their subjective complaints, and (3) evaluating abnormal intra-oral findings that are consistent with decreased salivary gland function.
6. Manage the oral health problems directly caused by salivary gland dysfunction.
7. Make an overall positive impact in the life of a patient with xerostomia (dry mouth).

HOW do I prepare myself to transfer this knowledge to patient care?

 Go to Chapter 43 content on your CD-ROM or search for "Saliva."

CD Exercises

- *43-1: Salivary Gland Dysfunction—Reference File:* Recognize the causes and effects of xerostomia. This exercise can be transferred to the reference file.
- *43-2: Dental Management of Salivary Gland Dysfunction:* Match the symptom to the most appropriate treatment for xerostomia.
- *43-3: Clues to Determine the Presense of Xerostomia— Ann Cronin:* Based on patient need and records, determine whether salivary dysfunction is present.

Textbook

Review Case Study 43-1, Dental Management of Salivary Gland Dysfunction, and the case applications.

For important concepts and application of knowledge, tables and boxes listed here may be especially helpful for clinical transfer and may be used as clinical resources:

- Box 43-1: Functions of Saliva
- Box 43-2: Oral Signs and Symptoms of Adverse Drug Reactions
- Box 43-3: Drug Categories that Cause Xerostomia
- Boxes 43-4 through 43-7 provide clues to determine the presence of xerostomia.
- Table 43-1 reviews the three major salivary glands.

HOW can I more effectively use this knowledge?

Critical Thinking Activities

Use the following worksheets to complete activities #1 and #2.

1. Visit five pharmacies, and determine the type of salivary substitutes each one stocks. Record your findings on Worksheet #1.
2. Ask the pharmacist at each of the five pharmacies visited what advice is provided to patients who have problems with xerostomia or dry mouth. Record their answers on each sheet of Worksheet #2.
3. Develop an educational pamphlet outlining the signs and symptoms indicative of xerostomia. Provide oral self-care recommendations for the patient with xerostomia.
4. Ask your personal dentist or dental hygienist whether his or her practice treats any patients with Sjögren's syndrome (SS) and, if so, how this patient is managed.
5. Obtain both stimulated and unstimulated salivary samples on two people and compare amounts. If differences exist between the stimulated and unstimulated samples, what questions would you then consider asking the subjects that might have an impact on the quantities obtained and the differences?

Worksheet #1

Record your findings from Critical Thinking Activity #1 in the following table.

	Pharmacy 1	Pharmacy 2	Pharmacy 3	Pharmacy 4	Pharmacy 5
Type of salivay subsitute sold					
Price range					
Side effect					
Suggested intake per day					

Worksheet #2

Use the following worksheet to record responses from Critical Thinking Activity #2. Ask the following questions and include two of your own during the interview.

Pharmacist #1

What do you tell patients in regard to the side effects and the daily intake? _____

_____

_____

_____

Should the side effects be a concern? _____

_____

_____

_____

Will the side effects negate the positive effect of the medication? _____

_____

_____

_____

Should the intake be altered according to personal circumstances? _____

_____

_____

_____

Individual question #1 _____

_____

_____

Individual question #2 _____

_____

_____

_____

Continued

Chapter **43** **Saliva and Salivary Dysfunction**

Worksheet #2—cont'd

Pharmacist #2

What do you tell patients in regard to the side effects and the daily intake? _____

_____

_____

_____

Should the side effects be a concern? _____

_____

_____

_____

Will the side effects negate the positive effect of the medication? _____

_____

_____

_____

Should the intake be altered according to personal circumstances? _____

_____

_____

_____

Individual question #1 _____

_____

_____

Individual question #2 _____

_____

_____

_____

Worksheet #2—cont'd
Pharmacist #3

What do you tell patients in regard to the side effects and the daily intake? _____

_____

_____

_____

Should the side effects be a concern? _____

_____

_____

_____

Will the side effects negate the positive effect of the medication? _____

_____

_____

_____

Should the intake be altered according to personal circumstances? _____

_____

_____

_____

Individual question #1 _____

_____

_____

Individual question #2 _____

_____

_____

_____

Continued

Chapter **43** **Saliva and Salivary Dysfunction**

Worksheet #2—cont'd

Pharmacist #4

What do you tell patients in regard to the side effects and the daily intake? _____

_____

_____

_____

Should the side effects be a concern? _____

_____

_____

_____

Will the side effects negate the positive effect of the medication? _____

_____

_____

_____

Should the intake be altered according to personal circumstances? _____

_____

_____

_____

Individual question #1 _____

_____

_____

Individual question #2 _____

_____

_____

_____

Chapter **43 Saliva and Salivary Dysfunction**

Worksheet #2—cont'd

Pharmacist #5

What do you tell patients in regard to the side effects and the daily intake? _____

_____

_____

_____

Should the side effects be a concern? _____

_____

_____

Will the side effects negate the positive effect of the medication? _____

_____

_____

_____

Should the intake be altered according to personal circumstances? _____

_____

_____

_____

Individual question #1 _____

_____

_____

Individual question #2 _____

_____

_____

_____

Chapter **43** **Saliva and Salivary Dysfunction**

DO I have all the answers?

Review Questions

Check your answers against the Answer Key at the back of this Study Guide to assess what you have learned.

1. Saliva is needed for all of the following functions *except* which one?
   a. Digesting
   b. Tasting
   c. Swallowing
   d. Sensing
   e. Speaking
2. Properties of saliva include all of the following *except* which one?
   a. Lubrication of the tissues
   b. Mastication
   c. Antimicrobial activity
   d. Oral pH regulation
   e. Debridement
3. The parotid gland is the largest of the major salivary glands. Which one of the following options is *not* a characteristic of the parotid gland?
   a. Produces 25% of total daily secretion
   b. Innervated by cranial nerve IX (glossopharyngeal nerve)
   c. Salivary secretion predominately mucus
   d. Salivary secretion predominately serous
4. Which one of the following chief complaints would you be *least* likely to hear from a patient with xerostomia?
   a. "My tongue feels like it is burning."
   b. "I have to sip water all day long."
   c. "Spicy food makes my mouth feel better."
   d. "Food doesn't taste good."
   e. "I have a hard time talking for more than 10 minutes."
5. Which one of the following dental management methods is best for patients with decreased salivary production?
   a. 1-year dental hygiene recall program
   b. Dietary management
   c. Aerobic exercise
   d. 3-month dental hygiene supportive care interval
   e. Use of electric toothbrush
6. Of the 200 most-prescribed medications in the United States in 1998, how many list xerostomia as an adverse effect?
   a. 50 to 74
   b. 25 to 49
   c. 100 or more
   d. 75 to 99
7. Salivary proteins serve many functions. Which one of the following salivary proteins contributes by providing lubrication and aggregation of bacteria?
   a. Sialoperoxidase
   b. Secretory immunoglobulin (IgA)
   c. Histatins
   d. Mucins

WHERE do I go for more information or support?

evolve

For suggested web sites and agencies, additional readings and resources, and more chapter-specific information, please consult your Evolve Student Resources. Because of the ever-changing nature of the Internet, please keep in mind that web sites listed and their content may change.

 CD-ROM

Reference files: As you work through the CD-ROM exercises, you should be able to print reference files and add them to your class materials.

The following exercise can be saved to a reference file: *43-1: Salivary Gland Dysfunction.*

HOW can I keep track of my progress toward competence?

As an ongoing picture of progress, record and monitor clinical experiences relating to Chapter 43 content in your Portfolio.

Self-Reflection

On a regular basis, review these experiences (with a faculty member). Identify strengths, weaknesses (not just numbers), and changes that you would incorporate into your clinical care plan now that you have had these experiences.

44 Neurologic and Sensory Impairment

WHY do I need to know about Neurologic and Sensory Impairment?

Dental hygienists will be caring for an increasingly older patient population with age-associated neurologic disease. In addition, medical science has enabled the survival of individuals of all ages with various neurologic diseases and injuries. Understanding the special needs of patients with neurologic disorders will enable the dental hygienist to provide safe, effective care.

WHAT will I be able to do with this knowledge?

1. Describe the prevalence, incidence, and distribution of selected neurologic disorders.
2. Identify the pathologic origin of each selected neurologic disorder.
3. List and describe the specific impairments that may characterize each selected neurologic disorder.
4. Describe the conventional dental treatment modalities for each selected condition, including surgical and nonsurgical approaches such as pharmacologic, behavioral, dietary, interventional, and using assistive devices and special accommodations.
5. Describe modifications the dental hygienist may need to make when providing care to patients with each of the selected neurologic disorders.
6. Describe preventive strategies, including chemotherapeutic agents and caregiver interactions, that may be needed for patients with each of the selected neurologic disorders.
7. Determine the most appropriate method of interacting with a patient who demonstrates a disability.
8. Identify the major legal implications for providing healthcare services to persons with neurologic impairment.

HOW do I prepare myself to transfer this knowledge to patient care?

 Go to Chapter 44 content on your CD-ROM or search for "Neurologic and Sensory Impairment."

CD Exercises

- *44-1: Key Terms—Reference File:* Select the appropriate definition for each impairment listed, and determine which part of the body is affected. This information can be saved as a reference file.

- *44-2: Deficits, Dependency, and Effect on Dental Care—Reference File:* Match the impairment to the oral care impact. This information can be saved as a reference file.
- *44-3: Deficits, Dependency, and Effect on Dental Care—Maria Bjork:* Based on patient scenarios, determine management strategies.

Textbook

Review the case studies and the case applications.

For important concepts and application of knowledge, tables, boxes, and figures listed here may be especially helpful for clinical transfer and may be used as a clinical resource:

Figure 44-1: Oral *sip and-puff* controlled self-powered wheelchair for patients with quadriplegia.

Figure 44-2: Custom-fabricated mouthstick for patients with quadriplegia.

Figure 44-5: Patient being treated in his own wheelchair. Note self-contained headrest.

Figure 44-6: Over-the-patient delivery system by A-DEC. (A-DEC, Inc., Newberg, Ore.)

Box 44-1: Grades of Skin Breakdown

Box 44-2: General Testing for Cognitive and Perceptual Impairments

The chapter is organized by categories of disorders that have similar pathologic origin and occur most often in certain age groups as laid out in Table 44-1.

Table 44-2 lists a number of conditions and deficits and their associated effects on the body.

HOW can I more effectively use this knowledge?

Critical Thinking Activities

1. Discuss the advantages and disadvantages of a custom-fitted mouthstick (as opposed to a *stock* flat plastic wafer type of mouthstick) for a patient who is quadriplegic.
2. Working in small groups of two to five, devise a hypothetical treatment plan to deliver dental hygiene supportive care services to patients with selected impairments with differing levels of severity. Have each group present its case and plan to the other groups for critique. Use either the specific disorders discussed in the chapter (e.g., stroke, autism) or the manifestations of such disorders (e.g., neuromuscular, respiratory) to guide your selection.

3. Arrange to visit a special needs patient care facility such as a nursing home, special needs day care facility, or behavioral healthcare facility to observe the techniques used in transportation and patient care. If this arrangement is not possible, then ask a professional staff member to address the class.

4. Work in pairs (one student as the provider, one as the patient) and role-play selected scenarios in a preclinical setting. The impairment selected for each student should be researched and presented by the student to the class before the preclinical exercise.

DO I have all the answers?

Review Questions

Check your answers against the Answer Key at the back of this Study Guide to assess what you have learned.

1. Your patient had a stroke 4 years ago and is stable but has difficulty keeping her mouth open for more than a few seconds at a time. In addition, her mandible occasionally moves involuntarily. Which one of the following options presents your best first chance to address these problems?
   a. Consider administering muscle relaxants to the patient.
   b. Refer the patient to a specialist.
   c. Obtain a medical consult.
   d. Use a mouth prop.
   e. Shorten the visit.

2. A patient with severe scoliosis related to spina bifida has scheduled a supportive care appointment. The receptionist noted that when the patient made the appointment, the patient reported that she had recently developed difficulties with decubitus ulcers. Which one of the following actions should you perform during this patient's appointment to prevent decubitus ulcers?
   a. Minimize the time the patient is seated in the treatment room chair.
   b. Ensure that the patient will freely communicate any positioning discomfort.
   c. Alter the patient's position to another comfortable position at least every 30 to 60 minutes.
   d. All of the above.
   e. None of the above.

3. You are about to treat a patient with a high-level (C5) spinal cord injury who has difficulty breathing freely. This condition is aggravated from a long history of heavy smoking before his injury and a resulting nagging and persistent cough. Your treatment calls for radiographs, debridement, polishing, and a periodic examination. Which of the following treatments is relatively *contraindicated?*
   a. Topical fluoride
   b. Rubber cup prophylaxis
   c. Air-polishing
   d. Subgingival irrigation
   e. Any of these treatments is acceptable.

4. You are planning to debride a patient's maxillary right quadrant. Because of the heavy deposits, patient sensitivity, and length of the last visit to treat another quadrant (more than 2 hours), local anesthesia will be used. The patient has an in-dwelling catheter and leg bag and takes *fluid pills* that his physician gives him for mild hypertension. Which one of the following precautions might you wish to exercise?
   a. Reposition the patient every 15 to 20 minutes.
   b. Check the leg bag every 15 to 20 minutes.
   c. Reschedule the patient for two shorter appointments.
   d. Avoid elevating the leg bag higher than the hips, and watch for kinks in the drain line.
   e. Treat the patient in an upright position.

5. You are disappointed that your older adult patient is not keeping up with her oral self-care, specifically her daily brushing and flossing. She reports that she "forgets a lot." Which one of the following options should you choose?
   a. Include a primary caregiver, such as a spouse or family member if possible, in the case and especially in the self-care instructions.
   b. Repeat the instructions several times.
   c. Ask the patient to repeat the instructions to you.
   d. Schedule the patient for bimonthly recalls.
   e. All of the above.

6. A patient mentions that she has had several operations, procedures, and medications prescribed in the last few years for cataract formations. Which one of the following dental procedures calls for special precautions?
   a. Radiograph exposure
   b. Administering local anesthesia with vasoconstrictor
   c. Full-mouth probing
   d. Air-polishing
   e. Using latex gloves

7. As you introduce yourself to a new patient and review his patient registration and health history, you become convinced that he suffers from dysarthria, possibly related to the loss of orofacial muscle coordination that you observe. The patient reports having been in a serious automobile accident resulting in brain damage and significant facial asymmetry and scarring. Which one of the following actions should you perform as a first step in effectively communicating with this patient?
   a. Ask questions that can be responded to with a simple *yes* or *no.*
   b. Give the patient a pencil and notepad.
   c. Speak clearly, and allow the patient more time to respond.
   d. None of the above
   e. Both *a* and *c*

8. You are assisting a dentist in designing and setting up a new dental practice that is located in a retirement community in your area. Which one of the following features should you stress?
   a. Access ramps for assistive devices such as wheelchairs and walkers
   b. Wider doors
   c. Handicap-designated parking spaces
   d. Dental chairs and delivery systems that allow for treatment of selected patients in their own wheelchairs
   e. All of the above

WHERE do I go for more information or support?

 evolve

For suggested web sites and agencies, additional readings and resources, and more chapter-specific information, please consult your Evolve Student Resources. Because of the ever-changing nature of the Internet, please keep in mind that web sites listed and their content may change.

CD-ROM

Reference files: As you work through the CD-ROM exercises, you should be able to print reference files and add them to your class materials. The following exercises can be written to reference files:
- *44-1: Key Terms*
- *44-2: Deficits, Dependency, and Effect on Dental Care*

HOW can I keep track of my progress toward competence?

As an ongoing picture of progress, record and monitor clinical experiences relating to Chapter 44 content in your Portfolio.

Self-Reflection

On a regular basis, review these experiences (with a faculty member). Identify strengths, weaknesses (not just numbers), and changes that you would incorporate into your clinical care plan now that you have had these experiences.

45 Mental and Emotional Disorders

WHY do I need to know about Mental and Emotional Disorders?

The dental hygienist will encounter patients with various emotional difficulties and will need to understand the nature of these difficulties to provide appropriate care.

WHAT will I be able to do with this knowledge?

1. Recognize certain behaviors associated with mental and emotional disorders.
2. Understand major classifications of mental illnesses.
3. Identify patients who may be at risk of hurting themselves.
4. Learn appropriate ways of relating to individuals with mental and emotional disturbances.
5. Know where to obtain additional information and make appropriate referrals.
6. Identify specific mental disorders and their relevance to dental treatment.
7. Develop treatment plans that include a mental health assessment.
8. Identify the major oral side effect of antianxiety medications.

HOW do I prepare myself to transfer this knowledge to patient care?

 Go to Chapter 45 content on your CD-ROM or search for "Mental and Emotional Disorders."

CD Exercises

- *45-1: Definitions and Classifications—Reference File:* Select the correct description, each disorder subtype, and distinctive modification of care for each condition presented. You will be able to save this information to your reference file.
- *45-2: Dental Considerations—Elena Guri:* Determine treatment based on patient need and level of distress for Elena Guri.

Textbook

Review Case Study 45-1, Fear and Anxiety in the Dental Patient, and the case applications.

For important concepts and application of knowledge, boxes listed here may be especially helpful for clinical transfer and may be used as a clinical resource:

- Box 45-1: *DSM-IV-TR* Multiaxial Classification
- Box 45-2: *DSM-IV-TR* Axis I: Clinical Disorders
- Box 45-3: *DSM-IV-TR* Axis II: Personality Disorders and Mental Retardation
- Box 45-4: *DSM-IV-TR* Axis III: General Medical Conditions
- Box 45-5: *DSM-IV-TR* Axis IV: Psychosocial and Environmental Problems
- Box 45-6: *DSM-IV-TR* Classification
- Box 45-7: *DSM-IV-TR* Anxiety Disorders
- Box 45-8: *DSM-IV-TR* Diagnostic Criteria for Panic Attack
- Box 45-9: *DSM-IV-TR* Diagnostic Criteria for Panic Disorder
- Box 45-11: *DSM-IV-TR* Diagnostic Criteria for Major Depressive Episode
- Box 45-12: DSM-IV-TR Diagnostic Criteria for Narcissistic Personality Disorder
- Box 45-13: *DSM-IV-TR* Diagnostic Criteria for Avoidant Personality Disorder
- Box 45-14: *DSM-IV-TR* Diagnostic Criteria for Dependent Personality Disorder
- Box 45-15: *DSM-IV-TR* Diagnostic Criteria for Obsessive-Compulsive Personality Disorder
- Box 45-16: *DSM-IV-TR* Diagnostic Criteria for and Types of Anorexia Nervosa
- Box 45-17: *DSM-IV-TR* Diagnostic Criteria for Bulimia Nervosa
- Box 45-18: *DSM-IV-TR* Diagnostic Criteria for Schizophrenia

HOW can I more effectively use this knowledge?

Critical Thinking Activities

1. Consider how U.S. culture views women in the popular media (e.g., movies, advertisements, fashion magazines). Do you share those views? What attributes do you include in your attitude about women's appearance?
2. If you had to develop a dental health plan for a mental health hospital, what would be the component elements of that plan? What parts of that plan would differ significantly from what you might expect to do in private practice?

229

3. Based on your understanding of the oral implications of the use of psychotropic medications, do you think that psychiatrists or general practitioners should inform patients about potential oral health problems and their prevention? If so, what information do you think should be provided? Should dental healthcare professionals alert the medical community about the effects of these medications on oral health?

4. Considering the prevalence of mental disorders, do you think the development of a mental health "screening" would be of value? What areas would you address, and how would you approach the patient on sensitive issues?

5. If you were to provide information to medical professionals (e.g., psychiatrists, psychiatric nurses, primary care providers) about oral care and mental health, what means of communication would be best? Given your recommendation, develop an outline of the program or presentation and review it with a colleague.

DO I have all the answers?

Review Questions

Check your answers against the Answer Key at the back of this Study Guide to assess what you have learned.

1. Which one of the following antidepressants is a selective serotonin reuptake inhibitor (SSRI)?
   a. Wellbutrin (bupropion)
   b. Serzone (nefazodone)
   c. Zoloft (sertraline)
   d. Nardil (phenelzine)
   e. Tofranil (imipramine)

2. Which one of the following disorders is the fear of germs?
   a. Acrophobia
   b. Claustrophobia
   c. Mysophobia
   d. Demophobia
   e. Haphephobia

3. If a person had a negative life event beyond normal experience and disruptive of previously held views, which one of the following disorders would likely be the primary diagnosis?
   a. Bipolar disorder
   b. Schizophrenia
   c. Obsessive-compulsive disorder (OCD)
   d. Posttraumatic stress disorder (PTSD)
   e. Major depressive episode

4. An individual who consumes large amounts of food in an almost frenzied state and then uses extraordinary means to prevent weight gain would be suffering from which one of the following disorders?
   a. OCD
   b. Anorexia nervosa
   c. Histrionic personality disorder
   d. Bulimia nervosa
   e. Dissociative disorder

5. A person who hears voices from outerspace has which one of the following symptoms?
   a. Delusion
   b. Hallucination
   c. Disorganized speech
   d. Catatonic behavior
   e. Flattened affect

6. Which one of the following is the manual developed by the American Psychiatric Association (APA) that names and categorizes more than 200 mental disorders?
   a. *DSM-IV-TR*
   b. *ICD-10*
   c. *NIDA*
   d. *NIMH-4*

7. Which one of the following drug categories would most likely cause tardive dyskinesia (TD)?
   a. Antidepressant
   b. Antianxiety
   c. Antipsychotic
   d. Antimanic

8. Which one of the following would *not* be a diagnostic criterion for a major depressive episode?
   a. Loss of interest in previously enjoyable activities
   b. Disruption of normal sleep patterns
   c. Sense of entitlement
   d. Significant increase or decrease in food intake
   e. Feelings of worthlessness or hopelessness

WHERE do I go for more information or support?

 evolve

For suggested web sites and agencies, additional readings and resources, and more chapter-specific information, please consult your Evolve Student Resources. Because of the ever-changing nature of the Internet, please keep in mind that web sites listed and their content may change.

CD-ROM

Reference files: As you work through the CD-ROM exercises, you should be able to print reference files and add them to your class materials. Exercise 45-1: Dental Considerations, can be saved to your reference files.

HOW can I keep track of my progress toward competence?

As an ongoing picture of progress, record and monitor clinical experiences relating to Chapter 45 content in your Portfolio.

Self-Reflection

On a regular basis, review these experiences (with a faculty member). Identify strengths, weaknesses (not just numbers), and changes that you would incorporate into your clinical care plan now that you have had these experiences.

46 Immune System Dysfunction

WHY do I need to know about Immune System Dysfunction?

Autoimmune disorders primarily affect women, who often experience one or more of these conditions throughout their lives. Most autoimmune diseases are treated with steroids that pose significant long-term risks to the body, including adrenal suppression. Invasive dental procedures and stress increase the risk for adrenal crisis, and patients may require steroid supplementation as a part of a stress-reduction protocol. Most autoimmune diseases have oral manifestations that require dental hygiene intervention.

WHAT will I be able to do with this knowledge?

1. Describe the pathophysiologic nature of immune system dysfunction.
2. Identify common signs and symptoms of various autoimmune diseases.
3. Discuss the classes of drugs that are frequently used to treat autoimmune diseases.
4. Identify oral manifestations of common autoimmune diseases.
5. Recognize the adverse oral complications associated with the classes of drugs used to treat autoimmune diseases.
6. Discuss the effects of chronic steroid use on the human body.
7. Describe risk-reduction strategies used in the dental office to prevent complications associated with adrenal suppression.
8. Implement dental hygiene management considerations for treating patients with autoimmune disease.

HOW do I prepare myself to transfer this knowledge to patient care?

 Go to Chapter 46 content on your CD-ROM or search for "Immune System."

CD Exercises

- *46-1: Understanding Immune System Dysfunction:* Given a diagnosis, match the anticipated clinical symptoms and the distinct modifications to care.

Textbook

Review Case Study 46-1, Suspicious History of Autoimmune Disease, and the case applications.

For important concepts and application of knowledge, tables and boxes listed here may be especially helpful for clinical transfer and may be used as a clinical resource:

- Box 46-1: Oral Manifestations of Sjögren's Syndrome
- Box 46-2: Key Health Messages for Individuals with Diabetes
- Box 46-3: Topical Corticosteroids
- Table 46-1: Drugs Used for the Management of Rheumatoid Arthritis
- Table 46-2: Signs and Symptoms of Systemic Lupus Erythematosus
- Table 46-3: Clinical Features of Scleroderma
- Table 46-4: Medications Used to Treat Scleroderma
- Table 46-5: Insulin Preparations
- Table 46-6: Common Signs and Symptoms of Thyroid Disease
- Table 46-7: Other Common Symptoms of Chronic Fatigue Syndrome

HOW can I more effectively use this knowledge?

Critical Thinking Activities

1. Interview a patient with an autoimmune disease. Ask the patient to describe how living with this disease affect his or her quality of life and ability to perform activities of daily living (ADLs).
2. Assess the ability of a patient with an autoimmune disease to perform manual plaque removal. Offer various devices to the patient, and ask the patient to demonstrate the use of each device. Make modifications to the existing device, or offer suggestions to improve technique.
3. Interview a patient with an autoimmune disease, and ask how the symptoms of fatigue and pain affect his or her quality of life. Ask the patient how he or she manages these conditions to improve the ability to function. List any medications that the patient is taking to manage these symptoms, and assess whether the patient is receiving adequate symptom control. Note any oral side effects caused by these medications, and recommend appropriate dental hygiene interventions to address these complications.

4. Identify those patients who are at highest risk for adrenal suppression, and describe how you would manage a patient with complications during periodontal or oral surgery.
5. Develop dental hygiene treatment plans for use with patients with different autoimmune diseases. Include risk assessment, oral and physical examination protocols, oral hygiene instructions, and practice management considerations.
6. Offer an oral health workshop at a local support group for patients with a specific autoimmune disease. Teach patients how their disease may affect the oral cavity and how they can improve their oral health. Offer a variety of preventive strategies for patients to try at home. Discuss various products and demonstrate techniques that patients can incorporate into their home care routine.

DO I have all the answers?

Review Questions

Check your answers against the Answer Key at the back of this Study Guide to assess what you have learned.

1. Which of the following triads characterize Sjögren's syndrome (SS)?
   a. Xerostomia, xerophthalmia, and exocrine gland dysfunction
   b. Xerostomia, exocrine gland dysfunction, and rheumatologic disorders
   c. Xerostomia, keratoconjunctivitis sicca (KCS), and neurologic disorders
   d. Xerostomia, KCS, and connective tissue disorders
2. Individuals with SS have a higher incidence of which one of the following?
   a. Pernicious anemia
   b. Hypothyroidism
   c. Hyperthyroidism
   d. Chronic fatigue syndrome (CFS)
3. Studies of patients with SS have demonstrated significantly higher plaque biofilm index scores and dental caries rates and increased alveolar bone loss. These increased risks are caused by either hyposalivation or the presence of autoimmune disease.
   a. Both statements are true.
   b. Both statements are false.
   c. The first statement is true; the second statement is false.
   d. The first statement is false; the second statement is true.
4. Destruction of the joint capsule causing synovitis and erosion of bone accompanied by deformity of joints and loss of mobility describes which one of the following conditions?
   a. Scleroderma
   b. Multiple sclerosis (MS)
   c. Rheumatoid arthritis (RA)
   d. Myasthenia gravis (MG)

5. Which one of the following is the most common oral manifestation of RA?
   a. Temporomandibular joint (TMJ) involvement
   b. Sleep apnea
   c. Pathologic jaw fracture
   d. Condylar erosion
6. Which one of the following is a classic sign of systemic lupus erythematosus (SLE)?
   a. Alopecia
   b. Malar rash
   c. Pruritus
   d. Vasculitis
7. Caution should be used in the treatment of patients with SLE. Prophylactic antibiotics are always recommended for these patients.
   a. Both statements are true.
   b. Both statements are false.
   c. The first statement is true; the second statement is false.
   d. The first statement is false; the second statement is true.
8. Patients with autoimmune diseases are often treated with supplemental steroid therapy. When providing oral health care, they may require a booster dose of steroids to prevent adrenal crisis.
   a. Both statements are true.
   b. Both statements are false.
   c. The first statement is true; the second statement is false.
   d. The first statement is false; the second statement is true.
9. CREST syndrome is common in which type of scleroderma?
   a. Morphea scleroderma
   b. Diffuse scleroderma
   c. Sine scleroderma
   d. Limited scleroderma
10. Oral hygiene care for patients with scleroderma may be impeded by which condition unique to this disease?
   a. Microstomia
   b. Widening of the periodontal ligament spaces
   c. Profound xerostomia
   d. Hypermobile tongue
11. Individuals with type 1 diabetes mellitus (DM) produce some endogenous insulin but not enough to manage the requirements of their dietary habits. Therefore insulin is the treatment of choice for these individuals.
   a. Both statements are true.
   b. Both statements are false.
   c. The first statement is true; the second statement is false.
   d. The first statement is false; the second statement is true.

12. Treating patients with type 1 DM during their peak activity of insulin may result in which one of the following?
    a. Hyperglycemia
    b. Hypoglycemia
    c. Diabetic ketoacidosis
    d. Diabetic coma
13. Which one of the following is the greatest risk with treatment of patients with hyperthyroidism?
    a. Myocardial infarction (MI)
    b. Epinephrine sensitivity
    c. Thyrotoxic crisis
    d. Stress and anxiety
14. The major difference between hyperthyroidism and hypothyroidism is that only one condition produces a goiter. Both conditions can be treated successfully with surgical intervention.
    a. Both statements are true.
    b. Both statements are false.
    c. The first statement is true; the second statement is false.
    d. The first statement is false; the second statement is true.
15. Which one of the following is the disease that causes profound weakness of the muscles of mastication resulting in a spontaneous dropping of the mandible and opening of the mouth?
    a. MS
    b. CFS
    c. MG
    d. Scleroderma

WHERE do I go for more information or support?

 evolve

For suggested web sites and agencies, additional readings and resources, and more chapter-specific information, please consult your Evolve Student Resources. Because of the ever-changing nature of the Internet, please keep in mind that web sites listed and their content may change.

CD-ROM

Reference files: As you work through the CD-ROM exercises, you should be able to print reference files and add them to your class materials. No specific reference files apply to this chapter.

HOW can I keep track of my progress toward competence?

As an ongoing picture of progress, record and monitor clinical experiences relating to Chapter 46 content in your Portfolio.

Self-Reflection

On a regular basis, review these experiences (with a faculty member). Identify strengths, weaknesses (not just numbers), and changes that you would incorporate into your clinical care plan now that you have had these experiences.

47 HIV and AIDS

WHY do I need to know about HIV and AIDS?

As a disease of significant concern and impact, everyone must understand human immunodeficiency virus (HIV) and acquired immunodeficiency syndrome (AIDS). More importantly, as healthcare providers, dental hygienists must understand and recognize the oral manifestations, infection-control implications, and postexposure management associated with HIV disease.

WHAT will I be able to do with this knowledge?

1. Discuss the etiologic factors of HIV and AIDS.
2. Demonstrate an appreciation and understanding for the epidemiologic mechanisms of HIV and AIDS.
3. Relate the forms of prevention for HIV.
4. Compare and contrast the clinical characteristics of HIV and AIDS.
5. Develop a care plan for patients with HIV and AIDS.

HOW do I prepare myself to transfer this knowledge to patient care?

 Go to Chapter 47 content on your CD-ROM or search for "HIV/AIDS."

CD Exercises

■ *47-1: Oral Manifestations of Human Immunodeficiency Virus Disease:* Given a distinct oral manifestation, match the photograph and the distinct modification to care.

Textbook

Review Case Study 47-1, Clinical Presentations of HIV, and the case applications. After reading the chapter, discuss the following:

All of the symptoms that this person exhibited at the initial visit were consistent with HIV seroconversion illness.

For important concepts and application of knowledge, review figures and boxed sections in the chapter.

HOW can I more effectively use this knowledge?

Critical Thinking Activities

1. Develop a plan of care for a patient with HIV who also has the following:
   a. Necrotizing ulcerative periodontitis
   b. Herpes zoster

c. Oral hairy leukoplakia
   d. Salivary gland dysfunction and xerostomia
   e. Recurrent aphthous ulcers
2. Evaluate each of the care plans developed on the previously mentioned conditions to determine whether interactions or complications may occur from multiple-symptom treatment recommendations.
3. Visit a clinic that provides care for patients with HIV or AIDS.
4. Present an educational program about oral care to a group of patients with HIV/AIDS.
5. Arrange to perform an oral assessment on a newly diagnosed patient with HIV and one with full-blown AIDS.

DO I have all the answers?

Review Questions

Check your answers against the Answer Key at the back of this Study Guide to assess what you have learned.

1. Which one of the following is a characteristic of HIV?
   a. It is responsible for causing hepatitis B.
   b. It is a deoxyribonucleic acid (DNA) virus.
   c. It is a ribonucleic acid (RNA) virus.
2. HIV is characterized by which of the following?
   a. A deterioration of the immune system
   b. A decrease in CD4+ cells
   c. Detection of p24 antigen
   d. All of the above
3. Which one of the following is the most common fungal infection seen in association with HIV/AIDS?
   a. Oral hairy leukoplakia
   b. Aphthous ulcers
   c. Kaposi's sarcoma
   d. Candidiasis
4. Which one of the following oral diseases has increased in the highly active antiretroviral therapy (HAART) era?
   a. Oral ulcerative disease
   b. Kaposi's sarcoma
   c. Oral warts
   d. Candidiasis
5. Oral ulcers that appear on nonfixed or nonkeratinized tissues are most likely which one of the following?
   a. Aphthous ulcers
   b. Ulcers caused by herpes simplex virus (HSV)
   c. Ulcers caused by cytomegalovirus (CMV)
   d. Traumatic ulcers

235

6. Standard precautions apply to all body fluids *except* one. Which one is this *exception?*
   a. Saliva
   b. Sweat
   c. Tears
   d. Blood
7. Biofilms in untreated dental waterlines are generally which one of the following?
   a. Highly pathogenic
   b. Not pathogenic
   c. Opportunistic
   d. Moderately pathogenic
8. Effective methods of waterline biofilm control include which one of the following?
   a. Flushing with water
   b. Chemical treatments
   c. Filter
   d. A combination of methods
9. Irrigants used in connection with surgical procedures should be which one of the following?
   a. Clean
   b. Aseptic
   c. Distilled
   d. Sterile
10. In which decade did the hepatis B virus (HBV) vaccine become widely available?
    a. 1970s
    b. 1980s
    c. 1990s
    d. 2000s
11. Unvaccinated (susceptible) healthcare providers exposed to rubella should be excluded from duty for how long?
    a. From the seventh day after first exposure through the twenty-first day after last exposure
    b. Until 24 hours after adequate treatment is started
    c. Until all lesions dry and crust
    d. Until acute symptoms resolve
12. Unvaccinated (susceptible) healthcare providers exposed to mumps should be excluded from duty for how long?
    a. Until 24 hours after start of effective therapy
    b. Until days after onset of parotitis
    c. From the twelfth day after first exposure through the twenty-sixth day after last exposure, or until 9 days after onset of parotitis
    d. Until 5 days after the start of effective antibiotic therapy

13. HIV is a disability protected by which of the following?
    a. The Americans with Disabilities Act
    b. The Rehabilitation Act of 1973
    c. State laws
    d. All of the above
    e. *a* and *b* only
14. A dental healthcare provider who is not comfortable treating a person with HIV may refer him or her to another provider. True or false?
15. Universal precautions are not considered a modification in practice under the Direct Threat Defense of the American's with Disabilities Act. True or false?

WHERE do I go for more information or support?

evolve

For suggested web sites and agencies, additional readings and resources, and more chapter-specific information, please consult your Evolve Student Resources. Because of the ever-changing nature of the Internet, please keep in mind that web sites listed and their content may change.

CD-ROM

Reference files: As you work through the CD-ROM exercises, you should be able to print reference files and add them to your class materials. No specific reference files apply to this chapter.

HOW can I keep track of my progress toward competence?

As an ongoing picture of progress, record and monitor clinical experiences relating to Chapter 47 content in your Portfolio.

Self-Reflection

On a regular basis, review these experiences (with a faculty member). Identify strengths, weaknesses (not just numbers), and changes that you would incorporate into your clinical care plan now that you have had these experiences.

48 Cancer and Treatment Effects on the Oral Cavity

WHY do I need to know about Cancer and Treatment Effects on the Oral Cavity?

Local and regional cancers involving the head and neck and systemic cancers such as leukemia are particularly relevant to the dental hygienist because both the disease and the treatment modalities (surgery, radiation, chemotherapy, and transplantation) adversely affect the oral soft and hard tissues. The dental hygienist must thoroughly evaluate the patient's medical history, determine the appropriate precautions that must be taken before dental treatment, recognize oral complications of the disease and its treatment, and provide palliative measures to alleviate oral pain and discomfort; eliminate any potential sources of oral infection; and instruct the patient, caregiver, or both in appropriate home care to promote healing and prevent further complications.

WHAT will I be able to do with this knowledge?

1. Know the incidence and contributing factors of cancer.
2. Understand the terminology associated with head and neck cancer, radiation therapy, leukemia, chemotherapy, and bone marrow transplantation.
3. Understand the potential etiologies or risk factors of cancer, particularly those affecting the head and neck.
4. Identify head and neck cancer by its appearance, symptoms, and location, and be able to identify the stage of the disease.
5. Describe the early signs and symptoms of leukemia.
6. Identify the types of leukemia.
7. Discuss the various methods for evaluating head and neck lesions.
8. Explain the types of radiation therapy and the dosage regimens.
9. Identify the drug categories used in chemotherapy regimens.
10. Describe the process and types of bone marrow transplantation.
11. Describe the types of oral complications associated with radiation therapy and chemotherapy and their management.
12. Outline a typical oral care protocol for patients before, during, and after radiation therapy, chemotherapy, or both.

HOW do I prepare myself to transfer this knowledge to patient care?

 Go to Chapter 48 content on your CD-ROM or search for "Cancer."

CD Exercises

- *48-1: Dental Considerations:* Locate and label common oral caner sites.
- *48-2: Staging:* Determine notations used for tumor classification.
- *48-3: Radiation Therapy:* Match description and management of radiation therapy to the oral complication.
- *48-4: Radiation Therapy—George Burkett:* Based on scenario and patient record, determine needs for George Burkett.
- *48-5: Chemotherapy:* Determine management strategies.

Textbook

Review the case studies and the related case applications.

For important concepts and application of knowledge, tables, boxes, and figures listed here may be especially helpful for clinical transfer and may be used as clinical resources:

- Box 48-1: International TNM System of Classification and Staging of Oral Carcinomas
- Box 48-2: Self-Examination Procedures for Oral Cancer
- Table 48-1: Degree of Organ Radiosensitivity
- Figure 48-1: Relative risk of cancer related to alcohol consumption and tobacco use.
- Figure 48-2: Shaded area shows the location of most oral cancers.
- Figure 48-3: Lymph nodes of the head and neck.
- Figure 48-4: Oral mucositis in a patient receiving radiation therapy for cancer of the head and neck.
- Figure 48-5: Radiograph showing *radiation caries,* the pattern of cervical decay that can develop in a patient with xerostomia that occurs secondary to irradiation of the salivary glands.
- Figure 48-6: Advanced dental caries 2 years after radiation therapy in a noncompliant patient.
- Figure 48-7: Effects of severe radiation-induced xerostomia on the tongue and other oral soft tissues.

- Figure 48-8: Oral candidiasis affecting the palatal mucosa in a patient undergoing radiation therapy for a tumor of the head and neck.
- Figure 48-9: Skin erythema from exposure to therapeutic doses of radiation.

HOW do I perform these skills?

evolve

A printable version of this checklist is available on your Evolve Student Resources.

To provide a thorough evaluation of patients with head and neck cancer, I will:

☐ Identify the various methods for evaluating lesions.

☐ Identify head and neck cancer.

☐ Identify the stage of the disease.

☐ Describe the types of oral complications associated with radiation therapy.

☐ Discuss course of radiation therapy with patient.

☐ Identify oral effects of radiation.

☐ Set monthly evaluation appointments.

☐ Evaluate oral tissues at each evaluation appointment.

☐ Recommend appropriate palliative therapy.

☐ Set appropriate supportive care reevaluation appointments at conclusion of actual radiation therapy.

☐ Document all findings and recommendations in patient chart.

HOW can I more effectively use this knowledge?

Critical Thinking Activities

Use the following worksheet to complete activity #2.

1. Perform an oral examination on a patient with cancer of the head and neck area.
2. Visit a hospital radiation therapy department and observe the administration of radiation therapy to a patient with a carcinoma of the head and neck. Use Worksheet #1 to complete this activity.
3. Perform oral debridement on a patient undergoing radiation therapy for cancer of the head and neck and on a patient undergoing chemotherapy.
4. Observe the oral complications associated with radiation therapy and chemotherapy, and provide appropriate palliative instructions for managing each of these side effects.
5. Attend a maxillofacial surgical procedure for treatment of head and neck cancer.
6. Attend a bone marrow biopsy procedure.
7. Visit a transplant unit in a local hospital, if available, and discuss with one of the nurses the types of oral complications commonly experienced by the patients admitted there.
8. Visit a maxillofacial prosthodontist to observe the fabrication of various prostheses used in managing facial deformities associated with head and neck cancer.
9. Fabricate custom fluoride mouth trays for a patient with radiation-induced xerostomia.

Worksheet #1

Oncology worksheet for Critical Thinking Activity #2.

Patient _____

Date _____

Type of cancer being treated _____

TREATMENT INFORMATION

Name of medical or radiation oncologist _____

Information regarding surgeries (type, date) _____

Chemotherapy regimen (drugs, frequency, route
   of administration) _____

Radiation therapy (site of therapy, date of initiation) _____

_____

ORAL CONCERNS

Specific Oral Concerns for Therapeutic Intervention

Strategies for maintaining oral hygiene status _____

Supportive care frequency recommendations _____

Current dental condition _____

_____

EDUCATIONAL ELEMENTS

Current oral status _____

Anticipated oral effects of cancer therapy _____

Resources for family or caregivers _____

Referral needs _____

PATIENT ADVOCACY

List ways in which you might serve as a liaison
   among patient, oncologist, and dentist before,
   during, and after cancer therapy. _____

_____

_____

Continued

Chapter **48** **Cancer and Treatment Effects on the Oral Cavity**

POTENTIAL ORAL COMPLICATIONS

Condition	Symptoms	Protocol to Advise
Oral mucositis	Inflamed mucosal lining can cause a burning sensation. Painful ulcerations can make eating, drinking, talking, even oral self-care difficult.	Provide a thorough oral cleansing. Recommend using a soft-bristled or ultra-soft toothbrush. Recommend using a fluoride dentifrice or baking soda and warm water if sensitivity occurs. Remove all oral appliances when sores are present. Discontinue any oral rinse containing alcohol. Avoid use of hydrogen peroxide. Apply any chlorhexidine product with a swab or toothette. Generalized mucositis can be treated with an over-the-counter or prescription rinse.
Xerostomia	Can occur in degrees from mild to severe during therapy. pH change can inhibit protective capabilities of saliva. Increased risk of dental caries, especially at the cervical area. Resolves after course of therapy.	Recommend artificial saliva, sugarless chewing gum, frequent sips of water, ice chips, humidifiers, a diet of moist foods. Apply fluoride in a tray. Recommend a diet low in sucrose. Apply calcium phosphate in a tray for severe cases.
Neurotoxicity	Chemotherapy agents can cause peripheral nerve damage. Symptoms can include bilateral tooth-aches. Patient may experience tingling or numbness in hands and feet. On completion of therapy, the pain subsides.	Provide palliative pain management.
Infection	Candidiasis is most often noted in patients with oral mucositis and hyposalivation. Patients with a history of herpes may experience a reactivation during chemotherapy.	*Candida infections:* Apply topical antifungal. Recommend that sucrose be avoided. Provide more frequent soft tissue examinations. Provide special care for prostheses to prevent reinfection. *Bacterial or viral infection:* Provide proper diagnosis. Provide organism-specific antibiotic or antiviral therapy.

Condition	Symptoms	Protocol to Advise
Bleeding	Thrombocytopenia can result from chemotherapy.	Monitor platelet count: When platelet count drops below 50,000 cells/mm^3, discontinue flossing. When platelet count drops below 20,000 cells/mm^3, stop all oral self-care. Recommend avoiding any activities that may cause bleeding.
Dysgeusia	Can be complete or partial. Bitter or acidic affected first. Salt and sweet may be affected as therapy progresses. Resolves in 2-4 months after radiation therapy. Can lead to loss of appetite.	Recommend seeking dietary counseling for alternative food suggestions. Recommend that a dietary supplement of zinc may be appropriate.
Dysphasia	Difficulty swallowing is not uncommon in cases of head and neck radiation. Can be complicated by xerostomia. Can result in eating and speaking difficulties.	Take smaller bites of food. Eat a soft to semisoft diet. Take frequent sips of water while eating.
Nutritional deficiency	Dysgeusia, dysphasia, xerostomia, and mucositis can lead to difficulties in eating, and poor nutritional intake can result.	Recommend nutritional liquid supplements. Caution to observe sucrose intake.
Osteoradionecrosis (ORN)	ORN can cause necrotic bone and soft tissue in the area of irradiation. Postradiation trauma, such as extraction, periodontal infection, or even an ill-fitting appliance can lead to ORN. Symptoms can show immediately or may take years to develop. Mandible is more susceptible. Radiation doses higher than 7000 cGy pose a greater risk.	PREVENTION! Provide dental treatment before therapy. Recommend that daily fluoride gel applications in well-fitting tray are essential for life. Provide more frequent oral supportive care therapy. Provide hyperbaric oxygen treatments before invasive procedures on irradiated tissues may be beneficial. Provide antibiotic therapy and surgery to remove bony sequestra if required.

Continued

Potential Oral Complications—cont'd

Condition	Symptoms	Protocol to Advise
Trismus	Fibrosis can occur to the muscles of mastication after irradiation and can result in trismus. Onset is typically 3-6 months after completion of radiation therapy.	Use a mouth block during therapy to avoid scatter radiation to the muscles of the face. Recommend daily isometric exercises to improve range of motion. Use mechanical stretching devices that are available.
Developmental anomalies	Depending on the total and fractional dose, developmental anomalies can occur from radiation therapy.	Recommend education for caregivers of child patient. Recommend long-term dental therapy. Recommend preventive therapy before radiation treatments. Coordinate of a team of specialists if necessary. Monitor fluoride therapy to prevent fluorosis. Address psychosocial issues.
Skin erythema	Can occur as early as the second week of therapy. Desquamation can provide a portal of entry for infection.	Shield the irradiated area from ultraviolet rays; do not use soaps or lotions on the area; and avoid extremes in temperature (hot and cold packs) on the skin.

DO I have all the answers?

Review Questions

Check your answers against the Answer Key at the back of this Study Guide to assess what you have learned. Questions 2 and 5 refer to Case Study 48-1. Questions 8 through 11 refer to Case Study 48-2.

1. Which one of the following options is the life span of oral mucosal cells?
   a. 3 to 5 days
   b. 5 to 10 days
   c. 10 to 14 days
   d. 15 to 21 days

2. Mr. Fitzgibbons is at greatest risk for which one of the following side effects of radiation therapy?
   a. Trismus
   b. Mucositis
   c. Osteoradionecrosis
   d. Bleeding
   e. Dysgeusia

3. The side effect referenced in question #2 would be managed best by administering which one of the following measures?
   a. Artificial saliva
   b. Hyperbaric oxygen
   c. Chlorhexidine rinse
   d. Zinc supplements
   e. Topical thrombin

4. Which one of the following forms of fluoride is *not* recommended for daily application?
   a. 1.23% acidulated phosphate fluoride
   b. 0.4% stannous fluoride
   c. 1.1% neutral sodium fluoride
   d. None of the above

5. Mr. Fitzgibbons has which one of the following stages of carcinoma?
   a. I
   b. II
   c. III
   d. IV

6. Which one of the following organs is the least radio-sensitive?
   a. Oral cavity
   b. Salivary glands
   c. Bone marrow
   d. Brain

7. Which one of the following oral complications is most frequently encountered by patients receiving chemotherapy?
   a. Ulcerative mucositis
   b. Xerostomia
   c. Osteoradionecrosis
   d. Dentinal hypersensitivity
   e. Dysphasia

8. Based on Ms. Clarkson's current blood counts, she is at greatest risk for which one of the following oral complications?
   a. Infection
   b. Trismus
   c. Bleeding
   d. Xerostomia
   e. Neurotoxicity

9. Ms. Clarkson has an acceptable neutrophil count for dental procedures. She would not require antibiotic coverage if she needed to have a dental procedure performed.
   a. The first statement is true; the second statement is false.
   b. The first statement is false; the second statement is true.
   c. Both statements are true.
   d. Both statements are false.

10. Ms. Clarkson's platelet count is too low for dental procedures. She also requires some modification in her toothbrushing because of her platelet level.
   a. The first statement is true; the second statement is false.
   b. The first statement is false; the second statement is true.
   c. Both statements are true.
   d. Both statements are false.

11. Which one of the following developmental anomalies might affect Ms. Clarkson in the long term as a result of her chemotherapy regimen?
   a. Partial anodontia
   b. Malocclusion
   c. Small stature
   d. All of the above
   e. None of the above

WHERE do I go for more information or support?

evolve

For suggested web sites and agencies, additional readings and resources, and more chapter-specific information, please consult your Evolve Student Resources. Because of the ever-changing nature of the Internet, please keep in mind that web sites listed and their content may change.

 CD-ROM

Reference files: As you work through the CD-ROM exercises, you should be able to print reference files and add them to your class materials. No specific reference files apply to this chapter.

HOW can I keep track of my progress toward competence?

As an ongoing picture of progress, record and monitor clinical experiences relating to Chapter 48 content in your Portfolio.

Self-Reflection

On a regular basis, review these experiences (with a faculty member). Identify strengths, weaknesses (not just numbers), and changes that you would incorporate into your clinical care plan now that you have had these experiences.

49 Dental Hygiene Business Practice Management

WHY do I need to know about Dental Hygiene Business Practice Management?

Dental hygienists have a unique opportunity to positively affect the experience of each patient seeking dental hygiene services through professional practice management. Understanding the economic side of a dental practice is important as one prepares to exit the educational program and become a professional dental hygienist. Dentistry is a business; if employed in a traditional setting, then the dental hygienist will be expected to contribute to the productivity of the practice. This chapter focuses on the following:

- Patient management including scheduling and appointments
- Marketing services offered by the dental practice
- Office operations that can increase productivity

Possessing an understanding of these concepts, in addition to clinical competence and appropriate communication skills, can improve one's value and marketability.

WHAT will I be able to do with this knowledge?

1. Incorporate positive word choices into my vocabulary for communicating with patients, staff, peers, and employers with regard to dental hygiene services and appointments.
2. Identify ways of enhancing the patient's perceived value of the services provided.
3. Develop periodontal protocols for a dental hygiene department in a practice.
4. Determine the number of dental hygienists needed to provide dental hygiene services in a practice with 4500 patients of record.
5. Identify patient needs through the process of a chart review.
6. Discuss the relationship of the dental office and the service provider (dentist or dental hygienist) with a patient.
7. Explain the benefits of using the oral hygiene fitness report.
8. Discuss mechanisms for keeping patients informed of the services offered.

HOW do I prepare myself to transfer this knowledge to patient care?

 Review the skills you have learned and continue to develop your individual Portfolio using the CD-ROM.

Textbook

Review Case Study 49-1, Poor Self-Image Because of Appearance of Teeth, and Case Study 49-2, Concerns with Dental Hygiene Appointment Management, and the case applications.

For important concepts and application of knowledge, tables, boxes, and figures listed here may be especially helpful for clinical transfer and may be used as clinical resources:

- Table 49-1: Comparison of Effective (Positive) Communication Phrases with Ineffective (Negative) Phrases
- Box 49-1: Anatomy of the Supportive Care Appointment
- Box 49-3: Examples of Communications One Might Have During Appointment Management
- Box 49-4: Criteria for Patient Chart Review
- Box 49-5: Methods for Keeping Patients Informed
- Box 49-6: American Dental Association (ADA) Codes
- Box 49-7: The Relationship between Parties Involved in Insurance Benefits
- Box 49-8: Supportive Care Reliability Analysis
- Figure 49-1: Medical history update.
- Figure 49-2: *Oral hygiene fitness report* (OHFR).
- Figure 49-4: Example of a computer-generated periodontal charting.
- Figure 49-5: Personalized smile evaluation.

HOW can I more effectively use this knowledge?

Critical Thinking Activities

1. Observe a dental hygienist in a dental practice for positive or negative word choices when communicating with the following individuals:
   a. Patient
   b. Dentist-employer
   c. Staff
   d. Peers (if more than one dental hygienist is present in the practice)
2. From the observations made in the previous activity, develop a summary of the interactions observed and make suggestions for improvement. Include your thoughts on how the communications affected or could affect the patient's perceived value of dental hygiene services.

3. Interview a front desk staff person in a clinical dental setting. Obtain the following information:
   a. How many patients does the dental hygienist have booked each day for one week?
   b. How many of these are periodontal patients?
   c. How many cancellations were there in that week?
   d. How many patients are in the practice?
   e. Are appointments confirmed?
   f. When are the supportive care appointments (SCAs) made? (Are they prescheduled at the time of the current appointment, or is a card sent for patients to call the office?)
4. Perform the following analyses based on the information you obtained in the previous activity:
   a. Supportive care reliability analysis
   b. Patient appointment scheduling and management protocols
5. Identify overhead for dental hygiene services for a month. Use the following steps:
   a. Develop a list of expendable supplies used during a dental hygiene supportive care appointment.
   b. Multiply the quantity of supplies needed and used to reflect the number of patients treated in 1 month.
   c. Determine the cost for these supplies.
   d. Keep (in a separate column) the cost of nonexpendable items such as hand pieces, powered instruments, and tips and inserts.
   e. Take the cost of nonexpendable items and develop a per patient cost for 1 month's use only. This exercise can assist you in seeing the number of times these items need to be used to recoup the purchase cost.
   f. Calculate the total fee charged for dental hygiene services during the month (i.e., gross income).
   g. Add the cost of expendable supplies for the month with the figure for nonexpendable items (i.e., partial overhead).
   h. Subtract the partial overhead from the gross income.
   i. Subtract your salary from the gross income to develop a gross estimate of profit. Note that other supportive staff salaries and benefits have not been taken into account in this computation.

DO I have all the answers?

Review Questions

Check your answers against the Answer Key at the back of this Study Guide to assess what you have learned.

1. Which of the following would be the most appropriate use of the 4355 (full mouth debridement) insurance code?
   a. Moderate supragingival calculus, heavy plaque biofilm, and generalized erythema with bleeding on probing
   b. Maxillary first and second molars and mandibular anterior linguals present, with heavy supragingival calculus that extends subgingivally, making it difficult to obtain accurate periodontal probing depths

   c. Both *a* and *b*
   d. Moderate supragingival calculus and localized 6-mm pockets with subgingival calculus
2. Mr. Johnson is scheduled for a 6-month SCA. Upon auditing his chart, you find that he has been non-compliant with recommendations for periodontal maintenance and radiographs, as well as untreated restorative needs. How would you help bolster Mr. Johnson's commitment to his oral health?
   a. Use an intraoral camera to photograph restorative needs and areas of periodontal inflammation to engage him in the examination process.
   b. Discuss only those treatment needs that his insurance will cover.
   c. Assume that he is aware of his oral health needs and will inform you when he is ready to proceed with treatment recommendations.
   d. Inform him that the office will refuse to see him if he does not comply with treatment recommendations.
3. What are some ways the dental hygienist can enhance the patient's perceived value of dental hygiene services?
   a. Involve the patient in the examination process by calling out the periodontal probe readings.
   b. Provide the patient with an oral hygiene fitness report (OHFR) at the conclusion of each supportive care visit.
   c. Show interest in the patient by remembering personal information such as family and work issues.
   d. All of the above.
4. Which one of the following is a characteristic of a highly effective dental hygiene department?
   a. Delivery of chemical antimicrobial agents on every patient
   b. Adoption of "watch and wait" philosophy so that patients will not feel pressure to comply
   c. Individualized treatment plans catering to each patient's specific needs
   d. Recommendation of whitening procedures for every patient
5. You are consistently running behind schedule with your patients. Which one of the following would be the best procedure to eliminate without compromising the patient's health or quality of the SCA?
   a. Vital signs
   b. Mechanical polishing
   c. Head and neck examination and oral cancer screening
   d. Full mouth periodontal charting

WHERE do I go for more information or support?

For suggested web sites and agencies, additional readings and resources, and more chapter-specific information, please consult your Evolve Student Resources. Because of the ever-changing nature of the Internet, please keep in mind that web sites listed and their content may change.

CD-ROM

Reference files: As you work through the CD-ROM exercises, you should be able to print reference files and add them to your class materials. No specific reference files apply to this chapter.

HOW can I keep track of my progress toward competence?

As an ongoing picture of progress, record and monitor clinical experiences relating to Chapter 49 content in your Portfolio.

Self-Reflection

On a regular basis, review these experiences (with a faculty member). Identify strengths, weaknesses (not just numbers), and changes that you would incorporate into your clinical care plan now that you have had these experiences.

50 Professional Development

WHY do I need to know about Professional Development?

Preparing for professional employment can be intimidating to recent graduates. Creating a resume and cover letter that a job seeker can submit for a position resulting in an invitation for an interview is what every prospective dental hygienist would like. This chapter will provide instructions on developing these tools and a portfolio for use during the interview. The dental hygienist is part of the healthcare professional team, and this topic, along with maintaining competence and methods for attaining continuing education, is covered in this chapter.

WHAT will I be able to do with this knowledge?

1. Assess values, philosophy, and interpersonal needs.
2. Develop professional goals based on values, philosophy, and needs.
3. Determine attainment of goals.
4. Develop a resume and cover letter for professional employment.
5. Prepare for an employment interview.
6. Establish a respectful working relationship within the healthcare environment and on a dental team.
7. Identify ways to empower yourself and others.
8. Maintain competence.
9. Develop an educational career plan based on opportunities for advanced education.
10. Gain insight into the various options available to pursue an advanced degree.

HOW do I prepare myself to transfer this knowledge to patient care?

 Go to Chapter 50 or Portfolio content on your CD-ROM for all of these exercises.

Portfolio Features

- *50-A: Values:* Complete a values inventory to help establish philosophy of practice.
- *50-B: Philosophy of Practice:* Create a philosophy of practice.
- *50-C: Interpersonal Needs:* Complete a needs assessment to help establish career goals.
- *50-D: Career Goal Setting:* Create career goals.
- *50-E: Measurement of Goals:* Establish current interest in career paths presented in year 1 of curriculum.

- *50-F: Portfolio:* Review competency experiences, determine strengths and areas for improvement, and develop goals and means of evaluation.
- *50-G: The Future:* Provide feedback on sections of the textbook and anticipate changes to future editions of this learning package.

Make sure your Portfolio files are complete on these CD-ROM exercises.

Textbook

Review Case Study 50-1, Embracing the Dental Hygiene Profession, and the case applications.

For important concepts and application of knowledge, boxes listed here may be especially helpful for clinical transfer and may be used as clinical resources:
- Box 50-1: Description of Maslow's Hierarchy of Needs
- Box 50-2: Creed for Relationships with Others
- Box 50-3: Methods for Obtaining Continued Professional Education Credits

HOW can I more effectively use this knowledge?

Critical Thinking Activities

1. Perform a job search on line for a dental hygiene position. Create a resume and cover letter for the dental hygiene position.
2. Establish three professional goals for yourself for the next year.
3. Develop a plan for how you will meet these goals that includes measurable outcomes as follows, for example:

   I will improve my knowledge of the relationship between periodontal diseases and systemic diseases by attending a continuing education course on this topic or reading at least one article on the topic each month.
4. Evaluate the effect of this knowledge on your clinical practice and interpersonal relationships with patients and colleagues.
5. Establish one educational career goal for yourself after graduation, such as taking a class or applying for a program to advance your degree. List the schools from which you are interested in seeking information, and make a timetable of when it will occur.

DO I have all the answers?

Review Questions

Check your answers against the Answer Key at the back of this Study Guide to assess what you have learned.

1. Which one of the following options would be acceptable for an interview?
   a. Wearing a mid-thigh–length skirt
   b. Wearing nails with polish
   c. Wearing flip-flops
   d. Chewing gum
2. An advanced degree may allow a person to do which of the following?
   a. Expand job options
   b. Develop research skills
   c. Gain confidence in job skills
   d. Gain new knowledge
   e. All of the above
3. Which one of the following aspects provides the foundation for the way we treat others?
   a. Interpersonal needs
   b. Philosophy
   c. Values
   d. Goals
4. Which one of the following options best describes the dental hygienist's role within healthcare?
   a. Efficient healthcare provider
   b. Direct-care provider
   c. Disease prevention and health promotion
   d. *a* and *b*
   e. *b* and *c*
5. Which one of the following options best describes the intent of the Portfolio?
   a. Retain documentation of continuing education for licensure.
   b. Retain documentation for evaluating continued competence.
   c. Maintain interesting cases for review and learning.
   d. Keep personal notes for review and evaluation.
6. Which one of the following options is the most effective way to empower yourself and others?
   a. Compliment others on their performance.
   b. Communicate effectively with others.
   c. Provide education about the relationship of oral and systemic disease.
   d. Keep track of assistance of others in the office.

WHERE do I go for more information or support?

evolve

For suggested web sites and agencies, additional readings and resources, and more chapter-specific information, please consult your Evolve Student Resources. Because of the ever-changing nature of the Internet, please keep in mind that web sites listed and their content may change.

 CD-ROM

Reference files: As you work through the CD-ROM exercises, you should be able to print reference files and add them to your class materials. No specific reference files apply to this chapter.

HOW can I keep track of my progress toward competence?

As an ongoing picture of progress, record and monitor clinical experiences relating to Chapter 50 content in your Portfolio.

Self-Reflection

On a regular basis, review these experiences (with a faculty member). Identify strengths, weaknesses (not just numbers), and changes that you would incorporate into your clinical care plan now that you have had these experiences.

51 Commitment and Vision

WHY do I need to know about Commitment and Vision?

"By altering its present course, the dental hygiene profession can assume leadership in the risk-assessment movement by embracing novel, creative approaches to research and preventive dental medicine."* Knowing what the profession needs to advance in delivering health care is critical to the survival of dental hygiene. This chapter should be read while asking the question, *What can I do to direct the future course of dental hygiene?*

WHAT will I be able to do with this knowledge?

1. Generate discussion of trends and future directions for the profession of dental hygiene in the following areas:
   - Clinical practice
   - Education, licensure, and portability
   - Research
   - Public health
2. Identify the relationship of technology to the profession of dental hygiene.
3. Identify methods for staying current with dental hygiene research.
4. Discuss the role of the dental hygiene profession in access to care.

HOW do I prepare myself to transfer this knowledge to patient care?

 Make sure your reference files are complete on all CD-ROM exercises. (Use only on activities that will have reference files.)

Portfolio Feature

- *51-A: The Future:* Provide feedback on sections of the textbook and anticipate changes to future editions of this learning package.

Textbook

Review Case Study 51-1, Vision of Oral Care in 2020, and the case applications.

For important concepts and application of knowledge, the box and table listed here may be especially helpful for clinical transfer and may be used as a clinical resource:

- Box 51-1: Future Settings for Screening for Disease and Other Services
- Table 51-1: Using the Academic Model for Categories of Future Direction

HOW can I more effectively use this knowledge?

Critical Thinking Activities

Use the following worksheet to complete activity #2.
1. Working in a small group, research trends or markers for future opportunities in dental hygiene education, clinical practice, public health, administration, and management.
2. Projecting yourself to a future world of dental hygiene, imagine yourself at a conference with the authors from your textbook. For each of the following sections, what types of revisions or additions would you need to make as a result of *a change in technology, a change in educational requirements, or a change in the role of the dental hygienist?* Write your answers on Worksheet #1.

Environmental Ergonomics

- Which chapters would change the most? The least?
- Would the chapter on exposure control be more or less relevant to the future dental healthcare provider?
- Judging from the pace of change in workstation design describe your vision of the environment for delivery of dental hygiene care.

Anxiety and Pain Control

- Which of these sections would require the most revision? From what standpoint?
- Which of these chapters is more likely to be affected by changes in product development?

Patient Assessment

- Which chapters will require the most revision as a result of developments in technology? As a result of the potential role of the dental hygienist?
- Will the chapter on tobacco cessation be more or less relevant to the next generation of patients?

---

*DePaola D: Thinking big, *Dimens Dent Hyg* 3:10, 12, 2005.

- Will the chapter discussing the clinical manifestations of common medications need to be increased or downsized?
- What role will new technology play in revisions to the chapter on supplementary aids?
- Will additional chapters need to be added to this section? If yes, then what titles?
- Will any chapters need to be deleted from this section?

Care Modifications for Special Needs Patients

- Based on the Human Genome Project, which of these chapters will need the most revision?
- Would you advise expanding this section? If yes, then in what ways?
- Will any chapters in this section no longer fit under this section title in that these types of patient needs will no longer exist? In that these types of patient needs are no longer *special* but exist in most all patients who are treated?
- What type of active role do you see in the future in caring for the patient with head and neck cancer?

3. Using Chapter 50 as a guideline, develop a set of professional goals. Include a mission statement (about which you feel passionate in your professional career), a vision statement (what your role will be now and in 5 years), and specific goals. Remember that a goal is an accomplishment that can be measured in some dimension.

   Unclear goal statement: I want to be the best dental hygienist in the world. (This goal might serve as a mission statement, as long as the goal statements that follow can be measured.)

   Clear goal statement: I want to maintain my dental hygiene licensure by attending appropriate continuing education courses. I want to share my knowledge with my office staff within 2 weeks after taking a new course. (This statement sets a specific measurable goal.)

4. You have been asked to define the ideal dental hygiene educator of the future. What qualities do you believe will be necessary in assuming this role?

5. You have accepted the position as the President of the American Dental Hygienists' Association (ADHA). As part of the role, you have been asked to address all the incoming dental hygiene students for the year (5 years from today's date). Your message will be beamed by satellite into every school of dental hygiene across the world and downloaded to each student's personal computer or mobile cell phone. All students will hear your message at one time. What message would you like to deliver to them at this initial stage of their career paths? If you were able to tell them just one motivational element, one influence that has been an inspiration to you during your dental hygiene education, what would it be? What would you tell them to expect for their futures?

6. You have been charged with identifying the top five journals that all dental hygienists should read to stay current with the literature pertaining to oral health. List the five journals you would select, and explain your reasoning for choosing these journals.

7. List three ways to identify whether a journal is peer reviewed and based on original research.

Worksheet #1

Using this worksheet with Critical Thinking Activity #2, evaluate each of the following sections and note what types of revisions or additions you would need to make as a result of a change in technology, change in educational requirements, or a change in the role of the dental hygienist.

This worksheet is also available as Exercise 50-G on your CD-ROM, where you can complete it electronically. When you have finished entering your answers on the CD, save the file to your hard drive or a disk. Then send it as an attachment to: sjdnewcomb@aol.com

Environmental Ergonomics	Chapter Number	Yes or No
Which chapters would change the most?		
Which chapters would change the least?		
Would the chapter on exposure control be more or less relevant to the future dental healthcare provider?		
Judging from the pace of the change in workstation design from past years, will the future delivery be the way in which dental hygienists practice? What way or ways?		
Anxiety and Pain Control and Operative Therapies		
Which of these sections would require the most revisions? From what standpoint?		
Which of these chapters is more likely to be affected by changes in product development?		
Patient Assessment		
Which chapters will require the most revisions as a result of developments in technology?		
Which chapters will require the most revisions as a result of the potential role of the dental hygienist?		
Will the chapter on tobacco cessation be more or less relevant to the next generation of patients?		
Will the chapter discussing the clinical manifestations of common medications need to be increased or downsized?		

Continued

Worksheet #1—cont'd

What role will new technology play in revisions to the chapter on supplementary aids?		
Will chapters need to be added to the patient assessment? If yes, what titles?		
Will any chapters need to be deleted from this section?		
Care Modifications for Special Needs Patients		
Based on the Human Genome Project, which of these chapters will need the most revision?		
Would you advise expanding this section? If yes, in what ways?		
Do any chapters in this section no longer fit under this section title because these types of patient needs are no longer *special* but exist on most all patients treated?		
What type of active role do you see in the future in caring for the patient with head and neck cancer?		

DO I have all the answers?

Review Questions

Check your answers against the Answer Key at the back of this Study Guide to assess what you have learned

1. Which one of the following factors has had the greatest impact on the future of dental hygiene practice?
   a. Political association funding
   b. Patient needs
   c. Educational requirements
   d. Advancements in technology
2. The association between systemic and oral diseases is important to healthcare delivery, but the application of this knowledge should be in a private medical facility.
   a. Both parts of the statement are true.
   b. The first part is true; the second part is false.
   c. The first part is false; the second part is true.
   d. Both parts of the statement are false.
3. Leaders for future development need all of the following characteristics *except* one. Which one is the *exception?*
   a. Insight and commitment
   b. Vision and self-assessment skills
   c. Willingness to work alone
   d. Respect for others
4. Identifying systemic diseases may be as simple as obtaining a saliva sample, a crevicular fluid sample, or both. This concept and process can increase the value of the dental hygienist within the healthcare environment.
   a. Both statements are true.
   b. The first statement is true; the second statement is false.
   c. The first statement is false; the second statement is true.
   d. Both statements are false.
5. Which one of the following choices is the most likely set of characteristics required of an individual to effect change?
   a. Compassion and integrity
   b. Insight and commitment
   c. Energy and a sense of humor
   d. Organization and support
6. The National Dental Hygiene Research Agenda is:
   a. A list of items to discuss at a meeting
   b. The list of research priorities as outlined by the ADHA
   c. Important to the progression of the dental hygiene profession
   d. *b* and *c*

WHERE do I go for more information or support?

For suggested web sites and agencies, additional readings and resources, and more chapter-specific information, please consult your Evolve Student Resources. Because of the ever-changing nature of the Internet, please keep in mind that web sites listed and their content may change.

CD-ROM

Reference files: As you work through the CD-ROM exercises, you should be able to print reference files and add them to your class materials. No specific reference files apply to this chapter.

HOW can I keep track of my progress toward competence?

As an ongoing picture of progress, record and monitor clinical experiences relating to Chapter 51 content in your Portfolio.

Self-Reflection

On a regular basis, review these experiences (with a faculty member). Identify strengths, weaknesses (not just numbers), and changes that you would incorporate into your clinical care plan now that you have had these experiences.

Answer Keys

Check your answers to the Review Questions to assess what you have learned.

CHAPTER 1

1. **d** All of these components have changed in the last 100 years, but the need for better communication with patients is always present.
2. **b** Alfred Fones is attributed with having founded the formal dental hygiene profession. The other three individuals are important historical figures in the development of dental hygiene education and the profession, but they are not credited with the founding of the profession.
3. **b** More dental hygienists are employed in private general dental practices than in any dental specialty or other employment or job scenario.
4. **c** Modified *direct* is not a form of supervision identified in this chapter. Dental hygienists are licensed to practice under various forms of supervision, including *direct* and *general,* which this chapter discusses. *Independent* practice is another form of business in which a dental hygienist may work; however, this form of supervision is rare.
5. **a** Although all of the items listed have some association with oral and systemic health, the immune components are found in both systemic and oral health. These immune components are part of the body's immune response that maintains health.
6. **d** Dental hygiene programs are located in all of these institutions and must be accredited by the American Dental Association Commission on Dental and Allied Dental Accreditation.
7. **e** All of these items are involved in the evaluation and measurement of competence.
8. **b** Access to care is the greatest reason for changes in supervision and licensure. Alternative models for delivery of care to the underserved force changes in supervision.

CHAPTER 2

1. **e** All of the prevention methods listed have significantly reduced the incidence, prevalence, and severity of dental caries (see Box 2-1).
2. **c** Health is not only defined by physical aspects of disease or quality of life but also by *all* aspects—physical, mental, and social well-being.
3. **c** The Theory of Reasoned Action explores the relationship between attitudes and behavior. It holds that an individual's attitude toward performing the behavior and the subjective norm determine the intention.
4. **b** Knowledge is not the only determinant for changing a health behavior. Other factors play a significant role as well.
5. **d** Dental caries is five times more common than asthma, and it represents the single-most chronic childhood disease; it is not equally evident across all socioeconomic guidelines.
6. **e** All answers are true. The mouth is a reflection of general health and well-being; oral diseases and conditions are associated with general health problems. A profound disparity exists between population groups in terms of oral health; and many systemic diseases do have oral manifestations.

CHAPTER 3

1. **b** Nonmaleficence is considered by many authors to be the cornerstone of the Hippocratic oath. Nonmaleficence calls on clinicians to do no harm or act to remove harm.
2. **d** Separating the two principles of beneficence and nonmaleficence is not always easy. Beneficence calls on the clinician to act in the best interest of the patient; nonmaleficence dictates that the clinician do no harm. If the dental hygienist attempts to provide a service that he or she has not been trained to do, then he or she may harm the patient, and this action will not be in the best interest of the patient. Option **b** can also be considered the correct answer.
3. **c** Autonomy is the ethical principle that supports a patient's right to make decisions.
4. **b** The steps of the ethical decision-making model are to (1) identify the ethical dilemma, (2) collect information, (3) state the options, (4) apply ethical principles, (5) make the decision, and (6) implement the decision.
5. **d** Although informed consent may save a dentist or dental hygienist from an unfavorable judgment in a lawsuit, the true purpose of informed consent is to provide the patient with all material information necessary to make treatment decisions.
6. **b** Option **a** refers to contract law rather than tort law. For a patient-plaintiff to prevail in a lawsuit involving tort law, he or she must prove the following: (1) the dentist or dental hygienist had a duty to help (a professional relationship was established), (2) the duty was breached (lack of due care), and (3) as a result of the breach of duty the patient-plaintiff suffered actual harm or injury.
7. **c** The duty of a healthcare provider is to inform the patient (in terms that the patient understands) of the treatment; alternatives to the recommended treatment, including the risks and benefits of the alternatives; cost of treatment; prognosis of treatment; and risks and benefits of no treatment.
8. **c** A well-established legal precedent is that patients have the right to control decisions related to their choices of healthcare treatments. This is expressed as a right to self-determination.

9. **e** Documenting what, why, and how treatment was provided is important to communicate clearly to any third-party individual who reads the record. It is also critical that the individual who makes the entry have the necessary information to ensure continuity of care.

10. **e** Although dental hygiene licensure is a matter of state statutory law, dental hygienists are also bound by federal, local, and common (case) law.

11. **c** Although exceptions are increasing, most states continue to regulate the practice of dental hygiene through a state board of dentistry.

12. **d** To avoid malpractice, all healthcare providers must minimally meet a basic standard of care when treating patients.

13. **b** The dental hygienists may be violating the patient's right to confidentiality.

CHAPTER 4

Questions 1-5 require students to place the steps in appropriate order. The order is the application of the PICO process. First, a good clinical question is developed so that one can go to the second step of finding the best evidence. The third step is to critically appraise the evidence obtained and determine what is useful to answer the clinical question. The fourth step is to actually apply, or use, the clinical procedures or techniques selected. The fifth step is to evaluate the clinical outcomes of these procedures.

1. **c**
2. **a**
3. **e**
4. **b**
5. **d**
6. **e** All of these recognitions are important. The American Dental Association has defined EBDM and included the process in accreditation standards, indicating that educational programs need to teach EBDM for dental and dental hygiene practitioners to use these skills in practice. To have the American Dental Education Asscociation (ADEA) include EBDM in dental and dental hygiene competencies further underlines the importance in education and practice. Having journals devoted to EBDM provides students and professionals with the most current information on EBDM.

7. **e** All of the reasons listed except option **e** contributed to the need for EBDM. Effective care may have been provided prior to EBDM, but without EBDM adoption of useful procedures and research, findings into clinical practice were delayed. Practitioners typically continue to practice as taught in school resulting in little to no variation in practice patterns. For these reasons, EBDM was developed and is currently being taught and practiced.

8. **e** Based on the hierarchy of evidence from scientific studies, the highest level of evidence results from a randomized controlled trial. While other scientific investigations provide useful information, without randomization and controls as part of the research design, the results can be confounded by other variables.

Questions 9-14 require identifying characteristics that best describe two types of publications: Literature Reviews (LRs) and Systemic Reviews (SRs). SRs differ significantly from LRs in that SRs concentrate on answering a specific clinically focused question, narrowing them in scope to a greater extent than LRs.

9. **b** SR
10. **a** LR
11. **a** LR
12. **b** SR
13. **a** LR
14. **b** SR
15. The correct PICO order is **b, a, d, c.** This is a four-part question requiring the selection of appropriate terms for each part of the PICO process.
    P Main concern or chief complaint
    I Treatment under consideration
    C Alternative treatment
    O Measurable result

CHAPTER 5

1. **d** Clearly, options **a, b,** and **c** discount the patient's affect. Option **a** places Mr. Truman on the defense and assumes he is fully knowledgeable of the need for the surgery. Although option **b** considers Mr. Truman's emotional state, it labels his response perhaps inappropriately. Option **c** assumes that Mr. Truman is concerned about the potential pain involved in the surgery, which is also assumptive. Dr. Jones' empathy is indicated by the statement, "Mr. Truman, you seem to be concerned about the surgery." Although Dr. Jones is assuming concern, the response also allows Mr. Truman to comment further. This form of active listening opens avenues for deeper discussions of Mr. Truman's concerns, whether they relate to pain, cost, time, or other issues.

2. **c** Options **a, b,** and **d** are harsh and punitive. They will cause Ms. Buffington to respond defensively. Option **c** recognizes the time demand for flossing regularly. It suggests that Ms. Buffington is doing well and can do even better with more attention to flossing regularly. This response is far more motivating than the other three.

3. **d** Effective communication is far from a passive process. It involves both the sender and the receiver in a dynamic interchange. All senses are operating when communication is effective. Hearing seems to dominate the interaction, but subtle clues to the meaning of the verbal interchange are picked up visually.

4. **e** Note the use of "I" statements in this message. In this example, the dental hygienist is taking accountability for her professional knowledge and beliefs. Understandably, this is a difficult situation for the hygienist; consequently, *owning* the problem, so to speak, and using "I" statements is a powerful method to tackle uncomfortable issues. Although the other person may disagree, the message is clear. The dental hygienist is also being genuine, and the "I" message reinforces that value.

CHAPTER 6

1. **b** The primary function of granulocytes and monocytes is phagocytosis.
2. **d** Parasitic infections result in increased production of eosinophils.
3. **c** Mast cells primarily secrete histamine.
4. **c** White blood cells exit the blood vessels through pores via diapedesis.
5. **a** Uncontrolled white blood cell production results in leukemia.
6. **c** Chemotaxis directs unidirectional movement by neutrophils and macrophages toward the site of inflammation.
7. **b** Increased vascular permeability causes edema associated with inflammation.
8. **c** Molecules that initiate cellular signaling mechanisms and regulate growth, proliferation, and maturation of cells are known as growth factors.
9. **d** C5a serves as a chemoattractant for white blood cells.
10. **a** Leukotriene production is associated with bronchospasm and edema associated with asthma and chronic allergies.
11. **b** T lymphocytes recognize and destroy antigens from foreign sources.
12. **c** Cellular specificity allows the immune system to distinguish between millions of different antigens.
13. **b** Repeated exposure to an antigen results in a heightened immune response because of memory cells.
14. **c** IgG is the most abundant immunoglobulin in the body.
15. **a** Trauma to the blood vessel or surrounding tissues activates the extrinsic clotting pathway.
16. **a** Sutures are used to promote healing by primary intention.

CHAPTER 7

1. **a** Autogenous refers to self-infection as a result of introducing a microorganism from one area of the body to another. This includes the bacteremia induced during subgingival scaling and is a concern because it may cause infective endocarditis in susceptible individuals. *Aerosol* or *droplet* refers to the transmission of microorganisms incorporated into materials that become airborne from a host source to a person or another host. This can be either cross-infection or autogenous infection (back to the source); however, *autogenous* is the specific term used by definition. *Direct* refers to the transmission of microorganisms from a specific person or source directly to another person or host. *Indirect* refers to the transmission of microorganisms from a specific person or source to an inanimate object (e.g., contaminated surface or item) and then to another person or host. Because the microorganisms leave the host, indirect transmission does not describe self-infection.
2. **d** The dose or quantity of microorganisms transmitted is a significant factor. Some microorganisms are highly pathogenic in a small dose, whereas others require a large-dose exposure before infection is likely. However, if the host has a resistance to the specific microorganisms, then the risk of infection is reduced. Host susceptibility is affected by the individual's general state of health and ability to resist infection. This state can alter the affect of dose and virulence of the specific microorganisms. The virulence of a microorganism determines its pathogenicity, how infectious the organism is, and the conditions necessary for infection to occur. Virulence will have a significant affect on the outcome of infection; however, outcome can be altered by dose and susceptibility. After exposure and transmission of pathogenic microorganisms, each of these factors has an affect on whether infection occurs. Altering any one or all of these factors can alter the course of infection.
3. **b** A fungal agent causes candidiasis; viral agents cause hepatitis and influenza. Bacterial agents cause *Legionella* and tuberculosis; a bacterial or viral agent may cause pneumonia.
4. **d** Neither alcohol nor products approved for use as disinfectants are capable of sterilization. Some products approved as chemical sterilants can be used for disinfection if they are used according to the manufacturer's directions for that purpose. Products approved only for use as disinfectants are not capable of sterilization.
5. **c** Correct terminologies for hazard abatement strategies as defined by the OSHA bloodborne pathogens (BBP) standard are *universal precautions* (UP), *work practice controls* (WPCs), and *record keeping*. The term *universal controls* (UC) is not used in the BBP standard.

CHAPTER 8

1. **c** The dental hygienist worked in an environment that required her to reach for instruments, suction device, and air/water syringe. The stool was not designed for use as a dental chair. The entire work area was not ergonomically designed for dental hygiene procedures.
2. **a** Of the three syndromes identified by McKenzie, derangement syndrome is the most difficult to treat. With derangement syndrome, tearing of tissues has occurred and medical intervention is required.
3. **b** Three normal curves are found in the spine when in proper static alignment.
4. **a** The spine has two lordosis curves in the lumbar and cervical regions and only one kyphosis curve in the thoracic region. The two lordosis curves are convex toward the anterior of the body, and the kyphosis curve in the thoracic region is convex toward the posterior of the body.
5. **c** The operator's head should be between 12 and 14 inches from the patient's oral cavity. Any farther or closer positioning would indicate the operator either has not positioned the operator chair correctly or is leaning over the patient.

6. **d**   The dental light should be at arm's length for maximum illumination of the oral cavity. Arm's length is approximately 36 inches from the oral cavity.
7. **d**   Performance logic positioning is based on proprioceptive feedback; it reduces the times the operator has to change positions. Evidence shows that this positioning can reduce work-related musculoskeletal disorders.

CHAPTER 9

1. **b**   The design features unique to sickle scalers are its two straight cutting edges and pointed toe. Curets have a rounded toe, and hoes have a beveled toe. Files have multiple cutting edges, and explorers have no cutting edges.
2. **a**   Curets, in general, have rounded toes. However, a distinct difference between the cutting edges of universal curets and Gracey curets is that the universal curet has two *straight* cutting edges, whereas the Gracey curet has two *curved* cutting edges and only one usable edge.
3. **d**   Explorers have no cutting edges, and hoes have only one cutting edge. Sickles and curets have two cutting edges, and files have multiple edges.
4. **d**   Research has indicated that hollow handles permit improved transmission of vibrations to the clinician's fingers. The use of wider handles results in less finger fatigue because the grasp is lighter, which allows for improved instrument control.
5. **c**   Thicker shanks have increased strength, which prevents the instrument from flexing when heavy calculus deposits are removed.
6. **e**   In the modified pen grasp, the thumb and first three fingers have a specific placement on the instrument and a specific function to aid in proper handling and use.
7. **d**   A fulcrum or finger rest is considered a point of stability. Therefore a fulcrum is designed to control clinician and instrument movements.
8. **a**   The modified pen grasp requires the index finger and thumb to be placed opposite each other on the handle of the instrument. Because these fingers do not touch one another, they are responsible for rolling the instrument to keep the toe against the tooth when activating an exploring, scaling, or root-planing stroke.
9. **e**   To engage a piece of calculus, the face of the working end should be slightly less than a 90-degree angle to the tooth surface. This angle provides maximum cutting ability for the working edge to remove the deposit.
10. **e**   Scaling strokes are designed to be short and firm to remove calculus deposits effectively. By engaging the edge of the deposit, the clinician can effectively remove the deposit piece by piece, rather than attempting to remove the entire deposit with a shaving method. Overlapping strokes ensures the removal of the entire deposit.
11. **e**   An ultrasonic scaler is appropriate and often the instrument of choice for debridement.

CHAPTER 10

1. **e**   Sharpened instruments create an edge rather than a rounded surface. This edge enhances tactile sensation and calculus removal, and it bites into the deposit rather than gliding over it.
2. **b**   Instruments can become dull during treatment, rendering them useless for calculus removal. By keeping sterile sharpening devices readily available, the clinician can sharpen as needed.
3. **d**   Before activation, the stone needs to be positioned to create an edge when moved across the lateral side. An angle of 100 to 110 degrees helps attain that edge.
4. **c**   The stone must be drawn in small portions across the cutting edge to maintain the curvature of the cutting edge. If the stone is laid against the entire cutting edge, then the curvature will be lost and the cutting edge will be ineffective.
5. **c**   An edge has no surface and cannot reflect light. However, a dull edge has roundness and a surface that can reflect light.
6. **b**   By starting at a 90-degree angle, it is visually easier for the clinician to establish the 100- to 110-degree angle.
7. **e**   All of these principles are required to sharpen a hoe effectively. The hoe has one straight cutting edge that can lie flat against the stone. By angling the handle away from the stone, proper edge-to-stone contact is made to ensure the beveled toe is flat against the stone. Holding the instrument in a modified pen grasp with a finger rest ensures stability of the instrument against the stone.
8. **a**   Because the universal curet has two straight cutting edges, the stone can lie against the entire length of the cutting edge.
9. **b**   Only one cutting edge is used and sharpened on an area-specific curet. Therefore rounding the toe from the cutting-edge side is necessary.
10. **b**   An area-specific curet has a curved cutting edge. To maintain its curvature, the clinician should start the sharpening stroke at the heel and rotate around to the toe.

CHAPTER 11

1. **c**   Teenagers generally comply with healthcare recommendations if given a specific reason to do so. Because appearance is important to most teenagers, they are more likely to adhere to a healthcare regimen if the dentist focuses on an improved beauty-related outcome.
2. **b**   The healthcare model presented in this chapter was based on the biologic components of health and the influence that sociologic and psychologic issues have on the overall health status.
3. **d**   Oral health status can alter the perception of self either positively or negatively, depending on the patient's degree of health. If a patient's health is good, he or she is more likely to have a positive self-image. However, if a patient has significant disease, he or

she may have feelings of worthlessness, hopelessness, and general negative feelings about self. He or she also may feel out of control of his or her health (locus of control), which can have a negative effect on well-being. Clearly visible dental disease has a negative effect during social interactions. A patient may experience embarrassment, withdrawal, and a diminished sense of self.

4. **d** The core of anticipatory guidance theory is based on the need to anticipate patient needs. To do so, the clinician should understand the patient's particular life circumstances and know what events in the various life stages affect health.

5. **a** All of the other options can lead to early childhood caries (ECC).

6. **d** Nonnutritive sucking provides children with a means to calm themselves and to control self-regulation and emotions. It does not improve coordination.

7. **e** Dental disease can cause persistent dental pain and therefore make it difficult to eat comfortably. This can lead to poor nutrition if the patient eats only soft foods, which are usually high in carbohydrates and sucrose. In addition, dental disease often results in unsightly teeth, which may cause embarrassment in social situations.

8. **e** It is well proven that alcohol consumption, illegal drug use, and poor nutrition during pregnancy increase the risk of abnormal fetal development, including improper development of the teeth.

9. **b** Demanding a behavior change is ineffective for a patient of any age. Option **a** reflects the fact that adolescents generally are self-focused and desire attention. By listening to the concerns of their adolescent patients, clinicians can show that they are interested in them. Option **c** explains that by expressing an interest in an adolescent's life outside the dental office, clinicians can demonstrate to the adolescent patient that he or she is important and that others can relate to him or her. Option **d** shows that identifying something positive about the behavior of adolescent patients is a greater motivator than focusing on what they do poorly.

10. **b** Progesterone levels increase after ovulation, which results in changes in the endometrium in preparation for implantation of the fertilized egg and development of the placenta and mammary glands.

11. **d** Progesterone alters both the rate and pattern of collagen production in the gingival tissues, which results in a reduced ability to repair and maintain the structure of the gingival tissues.

12. **a** Enlarged, bluish-red, and distinctively bulbous gingival tissues characterized puberty gingivitis.

13. **d** Surgical procedures should be scheduled during the nonestrogen days of the oral contraceptive cycle (days 23 to 28) to avoid possible osteitis.

CHAPTER 12

1. **a** The essential elements of a health history are (1) patient identification (biographic data), (2) history

of past and present illnesses (medical history), (3) history of present oral condition (chief complaint), (4) family history, (5) social history, (6) review of organ systems, and (7) vital signs. A full-mouth radiographic survey is an important component of a comprehensive *dental* examination.

2. **c** Dull, constant pain in the upper right molar is a description of the patient's present oral condition or the chief complaint. The use of glipizide (Glucotrol) by mouth for diabetes mellitus (DM) belongs in the past and present illness portion of the medical history. Blood pressure of 180/98 mm Hg is a vital sign, and a 40-year history of cigarette smoking is part of the social history.

3. **d** Age is a component of the patient identification (biographic data). Alcohol use, emotional status, occupation, and level of education are components of the social history.

4. **c** A prosthetic heart valve has a high risk for the development of infective endocarditis (IE), and thus it is imperative that patients with this condition be premedicated for invasive dental procedures. A history of rheumatic fever (RF) (with no rheumatic heart disease) and functional heart murmur (HM) are classified as *negligible-risk conditions;* therefore premedication is not necessary for any dental procedures. A history of a myocardial infarction (MI) is not included in any of the stratified cardiac conditions for IE.

5. **d** The presence of *Mycobacterium tuberculosis* in the sputum indicates that this patient has active tuberculosis (TB). A positive purified protein derivative (PPD) means the individual has been exposed to the TB organism; a positive PPD by itself does not imply that this individual has the disease. A history of taking isoniazid for 6 to 9 months is consistent with the prophylactic approach for a person younger than 35 who has been exposed to the TB organism but does not have the disease. A negative chest radiograph denotes that no damage exists in the lung tissue. (TB would result in visible areas of lung damage on the radiograph.)

6. **e** Fluorosis is related to the ingestion of fluoride at levels higher than the recommended level for dental caries control. This can be caused by fluoride supplements or naturally occurring sources of fluoride. Xerostomia, candidiasis, periodontal disease, and dental caries can all occur in patients with diabetes mellitus (DM). These oral findings can be directly related to the metabolic and microangiopathy components of diabetes.

CHAPTER 13

1. **d** Xerostomia is the most commonly occurring drug-related adverse oral event. It can manifest as a quantity change, a quality change, or both.

2. **d** *Candida albicans* is of weak pathogenicity. It lives in harmony with other oral flora and requires local or systemic predisposing factors, such as immunosuppression, nutrition deficiencies, medications, xerostomia, and age, to produce a diseased state.

3. **c** Both topical therapy and systemic antifungal therapy are available to treat candidiasis. However, systemic antifungal medications may cause multiple drug interactions with commonly prescribed medications. In addition, resistant fungal organisms occur with repeated exposure to these medications. Infection with a resistant fungal organism can be life threatening to an immunocompromised patient; therefore systemic antifungal therapy is considered a "reserve" course of treatment.

4. **b** This history describes erythema multiforme (EM) and is likely the result of a hypersensitivity reaction to the sulfa medication prescribed.

5. **c** Indirect immunofluorescence reveals a distinctive histologic pattern that helps evaluate and distinguish oral lichenoid drug reaction lesions.

6. **a** Glucophage (metformin) is known to cause a lichenoid drug reaction.

7. **b** Phenytoin and nifedipine have the highest incidence of drug-induced gingival enlargement.

8. **d** Doses of phenytoin, calcium channel blockers, and cyclosporine are associated with drug-induced gingival enlargement, as are increased dental plaque and cellular changes.

9. **a** Hairy tongue affects the filiform papillae. It causes elongation, hyperkeratinization, and retardation of the normal rate of desquamation of the filiform papillae. This condition occurs anterior to the circumvallate papillae.

10. **d** Intramuscular (IM) epinephrine is administered next when oral antihistamines do not control angioedema. If that treatment is unsuccessful, then intravenous (IV) corticosteroid drugs and antihistamines are used.

CHAPTER 14

1. **a** Palpation is the examination technique used to examine the structures of the neck, lymph nodes, thyroid gland, salivary glands, tongue, muscles of mastication, and movements of the condyles. Auscultation is used to listen to the temporomandibular joint (TMJ) for crepitus or popping, to measure the blood pressure, and to assess for the presence of bruits in the carotid artery. Percussion is used to examine muscles, bones, and teeth. Probing in the dental setting refers to examination of the dental sulcus with a periodontal probe.

2. **c** The examination technique of palpation is used in examine the structures of the neck, lymph nodes, thyroid gland, salivary glands, tongue, the muscles of mastication, and for evaluating the movements of the condyles. Auscultation is used to listen to the TMJ for crepitus or popping, measuring the blood pressure, and assessing for the presence of bruits in the carotid artery.

3. **b** The submandibular lymph nodes are reactive when inflammatory or neoplastic processes occur in the salivary glands, lips, buccal mucosa, gingiva, teeth, anterior palate, soft palate, and anterior two thirds of the tongue. The structures associated with the submental nodes are the tip of the tongue, anterior floor of the mouth, anterior lower gingiva, and midlower lip. The jugulodigastric nodes are associated with the posterior tongue, posterior floor of the mouth, and maxillary lips. The mandibular nodes are associated with the mucous membranes of the nose and cheek.

4. **b** The submandibular lymph nodes are reactive when inflammatory or neoplastic processes occur in the salivary glands, lips, buccal mucosa, gingiva, teeth, anterior palate, soft palate, and anterior two thirds of the tongue. The structures associated with the submental nodes are the tip of tongue, anterior floor of mouth, anterior lower gingiva, and midlower lip. The jugulodigastric nodes are associated with the posterior tongue, posterior floor of the mouth, and maxillary lips. The mandibular nodes are associated with the mucous membranes of the nose and cheek.

5. **b** The thyroid gland is found in the midline of the neck and produces hormones that regulate the body's metabolic activities. Enlarged thyroid gland tissue may be clinically significant in the identification of patients with hyperthyroidism or hypothyroidism.

6. **d** The submandibular glands are located in the posterior part of the mandible and below the floor of the mouth (mylohyoid muscle). These glands are easily palpated even when normal. The ducts of the submandibular glands (Wharton's ducts) exit lingual to the anterior mandibular incisors.

7. **b** An infectious process results in an elevated temperature. The elevation in temperature then causes an increase in the heart rate (5 to 10 beats per minute for each Fahrenheit degree increase in temperature) and an increase in the respirations (2 to 4 breaths per minute for each Fahrenheit degree increase).

8. **b** Elective procedures should not be provided for patients with Stage 2 hypertension (180/110 mm Hg).

9. **a** Orthostatic hypotension is syncope brought on by a sudden change from the horizontal position to the upright position or by prolonged standing (peripheral pooling). Patients at risk for orthostatic hypotension are those who take narcotics, tranquilizers, or antihypertensive agents, as well as those with diabetic neuropathy or Addison's disease. Therefore the patient with hypertension should not be treated in the horizontal (reclined) position.

10. **b** All characteristics of the meniscus are correct except for option **b.** The posterior band of the meniscus can be displaced anteriorly in front of the condyle, and this condition will result in clicking or popping of the TMJ when the displacement is reduced (on closing of the mouth).

CHAPTER 15

1. **c** *Leukoedema* is an abnormality found on the buccal mucosa that appears as a white, filmy, corrugated surface. *Leukoplakia* appears as a smooth white film. *Candidiasis* is a fungal infection that appears white

and patchy and is associated with denture use. *Erythema multiforme* is initially a red-colored lesion that may ulcer.

2. **a** The *retromolar pad* is the area of tissue just distal to the most posterior mandibular molar. *Raphae* are located on the palate. *Tuberosity* is a bone prominence. *Buccal mucosa* is the internal lining of the cheek surface.

3. **d** After drying the surface of the buccal mucosa with gauze, normal salivary flow may be observed from the parotid and other minor salivary glands.

4. **e** Fordyce granules are associated with sebaceous glands, which are not located on the palate.

5. **c** Sublingual caruncles are located under the tongue at the anterior intersection of the sublingual folds and contain the *Wharton's duct,* which drains from the sublingual salivary gland. *Carabelli's cusp* is a lingual cusp of the maxillary first molar. *Stensen's duct* drains from the parotid gland and is located on the buccal mucosa adjacent to the maxillary first molars.

6. **b** *Foramen cecum* is located on the dorsal surface of the tongue at the apex of the sulcus terminalis. *Mental foramen* is located on the mandible. *Sella turcica* is a depression located on the sphenoid bone. *Median lingual sulcus* divides the dorsal surface of the tongue in half.

7. **e** The gauze and air remove excess saliva, which allows a clearer intraoral observation. A mouth mirror allows retraction, and an overhead light provides intraoral illumination and visibility.

8. **d** *Linea alba* is a white line, which appears parallel only to the occlusal plane, often associated with trauma. *Leukoedema* appears as a white, filmy, corrugated surface on the buccal mucosa that disappears when the mucosa is stretched. *Candidiasis* appears white and patchy, typically on surfaces of denture-bearing tissues. Candidiasis is also evident in individuals infected with acquired immunodeficiency syndrome (AIDS) or human deficiency virus (HIV). *Lichen planus* is a plaquelike lesion that appears more generalized throughout the mucosal surfaces and skin.

9. **a** *Filiform* papillae, the most numerous of the papillae, cover the dorsal surface of the tongue. *Fungiform* papillae are smaller, mushroom-shaped papillae scattered throughout the filiform papillae. *Circumvallate* papillae, which are large and distinct, form a V-shaped line at the posterior of the dorsal surface. *Foliate* papillae are sparsely scattered on the lateral borders of the tongue.

10. **a** Rugae are located on the anterior portion of the palate, just posterior to the incisive papillae. The palatine fovea are small depressions located anterior to the vibrating line. The vibrating line separates the hard and soft palates.

CHAPTER 16

1. **b** The patient's clinical examination reveals generalized accumulations of plaque biofilm and calculus

with accompanying pocket formation and bone loss, which are standard characteristics of adult periodontitis. She also exhibits increased spacing between her maxillary right central and lateral incisors, which indicates the presence of the disease for some time (chronic periodontitis).

2. **c** Occlusal trauma is a result of malpositioned teeth, including teeth not in occlusion, clenched teeth, and bruxism. This patient's health history should rule out pregnancy gingivitis and postmenopausal periodontitis. Aspirin-associated bleeding when probed is a result of chronic high doses of aspirin. Propranolol (Inderal) does not induce gingival overgrowth.

3. **c** When probing with 25 gm of force, a probe tip with a diameter of 0.5 mm will penetrate into the junctional epithelium in healthy tissue and through the junctional epithelium and into the underlying connective tissue in inflamed gingival tissue.

4. **d** The *2N Nabers probe* has a curved shank with millimeter markings, which allows access to and measurement of furcations. A *Moffitt-Maryland probe* is straight and unable to access furcation areas. The *explorers* may be appropriate for calculus detection in furcation areas, but they have no millimeter markings and thus cannot provide measurements.

5. **b** A Class II furcation involvement, as noted on the periodontal chart by the solid triangle, is a loss of bone that extends underneath the roof of the furca approximately 3 mm horizontally.

6. **b** Tooth mobility degrees 1 and 2 (as noted by the numeral printed on the crown of the tooth) are measured as movement in a horizontal direction. The numeral 3 indicates degree 3, which includes movement when the tooth is vertically depressed.

7. **b** Based on the patient's health history, her mitral valve prolapse with no regurgitation or audible murmur may be classified as a functional murmur. Functional murmurs do not require premedication, according to the American Heart Association's guidelines published in 1999. The patient's physician should be consulted to verify that the information provided by the patient is correct.

8. **d** To determine bone loss on a radiograph, the normal pattern of the alveolar crest must be identified on the radiographs. The normal crest of bone runs parallel to a line drawn between the cementoenamel junction (CEJ) of adjacent teeth. This line runs 1 to 1.5 mm apically to the CEJs. Any deviation in this line indicates some bone loss. The presence of radiolucencies is noted in the furcations of the molars, which indicates bone loss. Using the crest of the interproximal alveolar bone, the approximate depth of the bone loss is determined in the furca areas. (The radiographic images of bone loss show less bone loss than may actually be clinically present.)

CHAPTER 17

1. **a** Healthy teeth are not sensitive; the absence of a carious lesion does not mean that the tooth is healthy.

2. **a**   Use of the explorer for dental caries detection is less than 60% accurate; accuracy is closer to 42%. Relying on the explorer for dental caries detection can be misleading in the pit and fissure areas, can potentially harm the smooth surfaces of the tooth, can damage newly erupted teeth and cause cavitations, and can spread pathogens to previously unaffected teeth.
3. **c**   Attrition is tooth wear caused by tooth-to-tooth contact, and it occurs on the incisal and occlusal surfaces. An exogenous substance does not have to be present for the wear associated with attrition to occur. Loss of tooth structure caused by chemical action is called *erosion*. Abfraction is flexure at the cervical region of the tooth that causes mineral loss.
4. **a**   Abrasion is the process of tooth wear caused by movement of a substance across the tooth surface during cleaning functions. Chemical wear is called *erosion,* and wear not caused by exogenous material is called *attrition*. Abfraction is flexure at the cervical region of the tooth that causes mineral loss.
5. **d**   The initial fluorosis type of lesion is seen clinically as a white spot on the enamel, but these spots are formed from increased levels of fluoride during the formation process with no demineralization of the enamel surface. The initial white spot demineralization of the tooth surface is evident as a result of the loss of tooth mineral that produces porosities in the tooth surface changing the way light is reflected through the enamel. Infusion of exogenous proteins into the demineralized enamel surface turns the white demineralization brown.

CHAPTER 18

1. **b**   Bite-wing images require opening of the contacts of adjacent teeth. This area cannot be viewed clinically nor as well on another exposure.
2. **a**   When the primary beam does not open the contacts (which is achieved with correct horizontal angulation), the beam causes one image to be imposed over another (i.e., overlapping).
3. **b**   Silver halide crystals create the image in conventional radiography (as do pixels in digital imaging).
4. **d**   All of these are considered disadvantages of digital radiography.
5. **a**   Only cone-beam imaging technology provides a three-dimensional image.
6. **c**   This image is of a bridge (the contrast of materials indicates a porcelain-fused-to-metal bridge). A solid-gold bridge would not have the difference in contrast on the abutment teeth.
7. **a**   Answering this question correctly requires knowledge of anatomy. Although the mandibular tori and mylohyoid ridge are radiopaque, the location of these structures is elsewhere. The lingual foramen is translucent; therefore the radiopacity is produced by the genial tubercles.
8. **b**   If the packet had been placed correctly, the maxillary central incisors could have been centered on the film.

9. **a**   Knowledge of anatomy is again necessary to answer this question. The inverted Y seen superior to the maxillary canines represents the intersection of the maxillary sinus and nasal cavity.
10. **d**   All of these items would be considered when purchasing an intraoral photographic imaging (IPI) system for the dental office.
11. **a**   Both statements are true. The recommended focal length for clinical photography is 105 mm to provide a better working distance for the clinician and comfort for the patient. This distance also keeps the camera at an appropriate distance to maintain asepsis.

CHAPTER 19

1. **b**   A 3- to 7-day diet survey is more reflective of the patient's actual food consumption than the 24-hour record. A 24-hour recall does not contain the variety of foods that truly represent the patient's dietary intake. Evaluation of food texture provides only one tool by which dental caries risk can be evaluated. Evaluation of the type and frequency of carbohydrate consumption are also important to the dietary data collection process.
2. **b**   Nuts, fats, and foods that contain xylitol are noncariogenic and may actually assist in preventing dental caries (see Box 19-3). Saccharin, although noncariogenic, does not provide protection against dental caries. Raisins and peanut butter are retentive foods and may lower the plaque biofilm pH for more than 40 minutes.
3. **e**   Depression and diabetes are treated with medications commonly known to contribute to xerostomia. A liquid diet reduces the amount of the patient's daily chewing action; therefore if the patient does not chew as much, then salivary flow will be reduced.
4. **e**   Infants require proper nutrition to supply calcium and phosphorus for bone and tooth mineralization. Osteoporosis in older patients is an indication that they have experienced bone loss as a result of the lack of calcium in their daily diets. Alcoholics consume many empty calories, and they do not ingest a balanced diet. Alcohol affects the absorption and digestion of many nutrients. Pregnant and lactating women have increased nutritional needs. Their diet must be adequate to provide the essential building materials for the developing fetus or nursing infant and to protect and promote the oral health of the mother.
5. **a**   The frequency of consumption and the physical form of fermentable carbohydrates pose the greatest demineralization potential of a posteruptive tooth. Vitamins, minerals, and proteins provide needed building tools to teeth in the preeruptive state.
6. **d**   Although inadequate nutrition does not cause periodontal disease, optimal nutrition is associated with the host defense mechanisms. Therefore nutrition is a factor that influences periodontal disease severity and posttherapy healing time.

7. **a** The consumption of a fermentable carbohydrate causes a drop in the pH of plaque biofilm within 2 to 4 minutes.

8. **c** The consumption of a fermentable carbohydrate causes a drop in the pH of plaque biofilm within 2 to 4 minutes and can last for 20 to 30 minutes until the buffering capabilities of saliva return the pH to a neutral level.

9. **f** A dental hygienist should not try to eliminate all carbohydrates in a patient's dietary intake. Information should be tailored to each patient's individual needs. Nonnutritive sweeteners and sugar alcohols may not promote dental caries but can cause dental caries in patients with xerostomia. Both nonnutritive sweeteners and sugar alcohols contain a small amount of carbohydrate and, without the protective action of saliva, can create an acidic environment.

10. **a** Neutral pH of plaque biofilm is approximately 7.0. A fermentable carbohydrate lowers the oral pH to a critical 5.5, which allows enamel to demineralize.

CHAPTER 20

1. **b** Understanding each patient's unique clinical, biological, psychologic, and sociologic needs is critical to plan and implement appropriate therapeutic strategies. Prevention needs are individualized; however, clinicians do build from the knowledge base and increase patients' level of understanding that is appropriate to their needs and abilities. Meeting expressed patient needs can increase compliance; however, it is not the basis of appropriate care planning.

2. **d** Oral risk assessment holds to the principles of health promotion (see also Chapter 2) and, obviously, to the principles of risk and risk assessment. Based on findings, intervention and prevention strategies are designed.

3. **d** Although insurance coding is based on the therapy provided, a system-based gathering tool will not aid in predetermining which insurance codes to use.

4. **d** Patient assessment includes the review of *all* forms of patient data to complete the assessment phase of the oral risk assessment system.

5. **b** The concern surfaced in the listing of medications that can cause gingival hyperplasia, not because the patient reported a symptom or because the symptoms were clinically evident. This concern is further addressed in Chapter 30.

6. **e** Bleeding on probing is not a clinical evaluation tool for any of the listed conditions.

7. **a** The type of diet indicated in the patient example is most consistent in leading to an oral risk concern of dental caries. This information, coupled with the clinical and radiographic findings, indicates an oral risk concern (actual) for root caries and a potential for coronal caries.

8. **a** Although intervention and prevention can indeed be defined exclusive of each other, they can and do overlap in both the design of intervention strategies and the personalization of prevention strategies.

9. **e** Discussing the oral manifestations of current prescription medication is an example of personalization of a prevention plan, not of a therapeutic intervention. Remember, the patient in Case Study 20-1 did not have any oral manifestations from current prescription medications.

10. **b** Both the statement and rationale are false. Planning patient care *is* a complex process and is *not* built on the application of a standard that is routinely set for patients.

CHAPTER 21

1. **e** Personalizing patient instruction is the cornerstone of prevention strategy and is vitally important to both the patient and the clinician.

2. **c** The steps of the oral risk assessment process are *review, analyze, plan, recommend,* and *evaluate/reevaluate.* Step 4 is *recommend.*

3. **d** Reviewing all aspects of the oral care process is critical. These aspects are therapeutic intervention; prevention strategies; patient understanding, appreciation, and compliance; and outcomes.

4. **e** The only oral risk concerns for the patient example are an increase in plaque biofilm and gingival hyperplasia.

5. **d** Raising someone's awareness of an oral concern (a strategy) can occur through demonstration, discussion, example, or a variety of methods. For the case presented in the chapter, the patient needs to be made aware that the medication she takes has several potential oral side effects.

6. **e** The history and data provided for this patient do not validate any of the factors listed.

7. **b** Any therapy initiated should be completed to facilitate better wound healing, and reevaluation should occur as soon as possible after initial therapy.

8. **e** Any demonstration (either within the mouth or with a visual aid) that supports an understanding of the signs and symptoms of gingival disease meets this goal. However, pointing out areas of stain (that need polishing) does not speak directly to this goal.

9. **e** Although clinician satisfaction can be enhanced through the use of an organizational tool such as oral risk assessment, evaluating clinician satisfaction is not a measure or step in the system.

10. **d** All of these factors are important and must be considered in the personalization of the oral care plan to ensure optimal oral health. All factors, when evaluated together, provide the basis for the personalization of prevention strategies.

CHAPTER 22

1. **b** Calcium channel blockers, prescribed for persons with high blood pressure, can cause gingival hyperplasia, and this would hamper Mrs. Lightfoot's plaque biofilm control access. A controlled person with non–insulin-dependent diabetes mellitus (NIDDM) should exhibit no oral changes that would

265

interfere with plaque control. Naproxen, prescribed for Mrs. Lightfoot's osteoarthritis, should not interfere with her plaque control.

2. **d**   Gingival hyperplasia makes plaque biofilm removal a challenge and therefore can cause an increase in gingival bleeding. Options **b** and **c** are also likely to result in increased bleeding. Although clinical evidence shows that a change in diuretic medication would cause gingival bleeding, this option is the least likely of the four causes listed (and therefore the correct answer).

3. **b**   If Mrs. Lightfoot has no increased attachment loss, then the probe reading is greater because of swelling in the gingiva. Although probe readings may be greater in the presence of inflammation, an experienced dental hygienist should use appropriate probing pressure and angulation; therefore option **a** is not the most likely answer. Because her attachment level is currently stable, option **c** is incorrect. Option **d,** poor plaque biofilm control, is an incomplete response, because just the presence of plaque is not sufficient. The plaque must produce a change in the gingiva, which changes probe measurements.

4. **a**   Bleeding 16% or more should result in a 1-month shorter interval of maintenance care, so Mrs. Lightfoot should be seen before she leaves on her trip. If she is taking an extended trip, then option **b** is a necessary recommendation. Option **c** would lengthen her next preventive maintenance appointment (when the interval needs to be shortened). Option **d** is the least advisable, because this option is not based on the patient's risks or level of periodontal health.

5. **d**   Although all three other choices are good reasons for concern, Mrs. Lightfoot does not appear to be personally involved in her care other than maintaining office visits every 3 months. It can be inferred that her indifference to the maintenance procedures includes the instructions for her daily personal oral self-care. The reasons for option **d** may be many. For example, for some reason she may not have understood everything she has been told. She could have a language barrier or a slight hearing problem (or other sight impairment) that the clinician has not detected. If her teeth are sensitive, then she may not be able to accomplish her home care as well as she should. In addition, she may have inadequate time, support, or money for oral self-care aids (although she has faithfully kept her 3-month appointments).

6. **c**   Osteoarthritis could be why Mrs. Lightfoot's plaque biofilm control is not as thorough as should be expected. The hygienist should watch her technique; get her to talk about how much time she spends on her teeth; and observe and ask whether oral care is difficult to do with her fingers, hands, or arms. She may have misunderstood previous oral care instructions or have difficulty with manual deplaquing aids. If her diabetes and blood pressure are under control, then these illnesses would not hamper her plaque biofilm control efforts.

CHAPTER 23

1. **e**   All of the choices are appropriate methods for use in a case documentation. Among other things, case documentation could be used to educate peers, motivate patients, evaluate the outcomes of care, and provide third-party payers with information.

2. **b**   Of the three items to consider when developing a case (the purpose of developing the case, the intended audience, and the goal of the development and documentation), option **b**—intended audience—is the only option provided. When these three issues are addressed, the information or answers can act as an outline for organization, thoroughness, precision, and objectivity in the design, documentation, and presentation of the case.

3. **c**   Current and historical dental information is considered part of the patient profile (or patient information section) that provides basic information about the individual designed to introduce the patient to the audience. A complete radiographic series, initial clinical assessment, and extraoral and intraoral examination (EIX) are generally considered part of the clinical evidence section, whereas treatment strategies are generally part of the case management section.

4. **b**   Oral presentations are the most widely used case presentation format. Oral delivery can be presented (1) on a one-to-one basis, such as clinician to patient; (2) to small groups, such as a gathering of colleagues or patients; or (3) to large audiences, such as professional or public meetings.

CHAPTER 24

1. **e**   All of these conditions can occur from using the scrub brush method with a stiffer toothbrush.

2. **a**   Mrs. Cronin needs a large-handled toothbrush because of the painful arthritis and dexterity issues with her hands. She also needs a small head to accommodate some of the more difficult-to-clean areas in her mouth, particularly in the posterior regions. A small handle would not be appropriate for her.

3. **a**   The modified Bass method will allow Mrs. Cronin to cleanse under the gingival margin and to clean the tooth surface. Other methods are less likely to cleanse under the gingival margin.

4. **c**   The interproximal brush, although ultrafine, cannot effectively be used on facial, lingual, or palatal surfaces.

5. **a**   An important aspect of interdental cleaning is that the patient actually does it. Whichever works best, waxed or unwaxed, thick or thin, is of little importance as long as the technique is correct and the plaque biofilm is removed.

6. **d**   All of the options are correct. Toothbrushes do begin to show signs of wear within 3 months of use. If wear begins to show before that, then the brush should be replaced. The brush should also be discarded after any illness.

7. **b**   Based on the patient's tight contacts and rotated teeth, waxed floss would slide between the contacts with less breakage and shredding than unwaxed floss. Wood sticks and proximal brushes probably would not fit interproximally.

8. **c**   A soft, nylon bristle is preferred for every patient.

9. **d**   Because of the anatomical considerations in Mrs. Cronin's oral architecture, helping her properly angle the toothbrush to be certain the bristles reach the sulcular area would be the best idea. Ideally, using a sulcular brushing technique would be the best recommendation. Given her lack of dexterity, however, the next best solution is to observe and correct the toothbrushing method.

10. **d**   A powered brush removes plaque biofilm thoroughly and can be positioned in all areas when used gently.

11. **b**   The Fones method is preferable for a young child. Children do not have the dexterity or cognitive abilities to understand angulations or to perform the techniques required with more sophisticated brushing methods.

12. **c**   Studies indicate that most adults brush for less than 1 minute, and children even less. This is an insufficient amount of time to accomplish thorough plaque removal. The perfect answer would be to brush until all the plaque biofilm has been removed—no matter how long it takes. However, because most individuals, especially children, need guidelines, 3 minutes would be the best choice. The longer the child brushes, the more likely he or she is to remove plaque. If the child is using a fluoridated dentifrice, then 3-minute contact with enamel surface will help ensure maximal topical benefit.

13. **c**   The stiffness of the brush bristle has nothing to do with the extent of plaque removal. The soft bristle brush is tissue friendly and can be used in the gingival sulcus for plaque removal. The method of the plaque removal is important, not the stiffness of the bristle.

14. **a**   Because Peter likes to use a wooden toothpick, assisting him in its proper use is important to avoid tissue damage and ensure thorough plaque removal. Changing his interproximal cleaning method to one of the other choices may be counterproductive.

CHAPTER 25

1. **d**   Tooth mineral is a highly soluble carbonated apatite. The carbonate ion does *not* strengthen the enamel, but it makes it soluble to acids in the environment.

2. **a**   The hydroxide ion is substituted by the fluoride ion to form fluorapatite, the most resistant of the minerals to dissolution by acid.

3. **a**   Both statements are true. The actions of fluoride are both antibacterial and anticariogenic. Fluoride in quantities greater than prescribed can produce acute illness and even death if the quantity is great enough. The amount of fluoride in water supplies is regulated, as is the percentage and quantity in other oral care products.

4. **a**   Placing a restoration in a carious lesion is a surgical intervention to stop the dental caries process in that tooth only and with that lesion. The restoration makes the tooth functional again. The restoration does not provide a reduction in the bacteria responsible for dental caries development; therefore another intervention must be adopted to reduce the bacterial load for dental caries control.

5. **b**   The antibacterial effect of fluoride inhibits the bacterial plaque biofilm, and the anticariogenic effect is responsible for the decrease in the demineralization process while it aids in the remineralization process. Fluoride has no effect on stain reduction of the enamel surface.

6. **b**   Demineralization is caused by a low pH level of 5.2 or lower. A high pH level is not acidic but basic and is not responsible for demineralization. The teeth are constantly going through the process of demineralization and remineralization given the changes of salivary pH throughout the day.

7. **b**   Salivary proteins are present in the pellicle. These proteins and minerals consist of calcium, phosphate, fluoride, and bicarbonate that buffer acids. Antifungal and antibacterial components and immunoglobulins are also present in salivary proteins.

8. **d**   Small molecules and ions are driven along a concentration gradient by passive diffusion into the porous enamel. These ions and minerals consist of calcium, phosphate, fluoride, and organic acids. Demineralization occurs when the enamel is dissolved by the influx of the organic acids onto and within the enamel surface.

9. **c**   Saliva is correct because it is filled with not only fluoride ions but also with phosphate, calcium, immunoglobulins, and other anticariogenic and antibacterial components.

10. **c**   Dental caries is an infectious, multifactorial, site-specific disease that is transmittable from mother to child and is measured by the use of the Decayed, Missing, or Filled (DMF) index in the population. Dental caries cannot spread from the inside of one tooth (iatrogenically) to another site.

11. **b**   Dental caries is caused by several factors. Bacteria (streptococci mutans [SM] and lactobacilli [LB]) must be present for the carious process to develop. If these bacteria were present in one strain of animals when placed with the other group without dental caries, the bacteria were spread to the unaffected group through salivary contact.

CHAPTER 26

1. **b**   Controlled studies have been conducted on anti-gingivitis, anticaries, and antisensitivity agents but not on the development of periodontitis. Although gingivitis is a precursor to periodontitis, not all gingivitis turns into periodontitis; therefore controlling for effects is more difficult.

2. **c**   A dentifrice is in paste, gel, and powder forms because of the abrasive contents. A rinse does not have an abrasive effect.

3. **c**   Flavoring agents, detergents, and preservatives are the components within dentifrices that have been found to cause allergic reactions.

4. **c**   The Council on Scientific Affairs administers the American Dental Association (ADA) Seal of Acceptance.

5. **c**   The U.S. Food and Drug Administration requires manufacturers to provide evidence of no carcinogenicity and no allergenicity and proof of effectiveness for approval to market.

6. **b**   The type of group in which one product ingredient is compared with another is a *superiority study.* A large clinical trial of this sort is not a pilot study because of the study's size.

7. **c**   Stannous fluoride has been found effective in the prevention of dental caries, dentinal sensitivity, and gingivitis. It has not been found to decrease salivary flow.

8. **b**   The most effective anticalculus ingredient to date is sodium hexametaphosphate.

9. **d**   All of the salts listed are included in some antisensitivity formulations *except* sodium bicarbonate.

10. **a**   Nonperoxide tooth whiteners found in dentifrices are formulations of mild abrasives with a tartar-control ingredient.

11. **e**   Potassium nitrate is the most common active ingredient in commercial sensitivity control dentifrices. Other active ingredients that are used for sensitivity control include sodium fluoride, strontium chloride, sodium citrate, and potassium citrate.

12. **d**   True whitening dentifrices produce their effect by altering tooth color. For a whitening dentifrice to have the ADA Seal of Acceptance, the whitening dentifrice must demonstrate a change in tooth color by two or more shades.

13. **a**   Dentifrices with lower relative dentin abrasitivity index values are less abrasive. Therefore the higher the number, the more abrasive the dentifrice.

14. **b**   Sodium bicarbonate is effective in reducing oral malodors because it inhibits the volatile sulfuric compounds.

15. **a**   Xylitol is a naturally occurring sweetener found in fruits, berries, mushrooms, and birch bark.

CHAPTER 27

1. **c**   If the patient will comply with the therapy, pulsed irrigation is the simplest method of the options provided. Although Ms. Tevus would need to purchase a pulsed irrigator, pulsed water irrigation may stop the bleeding without any further intervention. Option **a:** Ms. Tevus can probably do more for herself at home to improve her plaque biofilm control. She is too busy to have to return to the office every 2 months, which also increases the expense of her care. Option **b:** Taking a culture is not indicted at this time. Option **d:** Nonsurgical care and daily good home care are effective on probe depths up to 5 mm. However, if her periodontal condition continues to worsen, a periodontal referral and a medical checkup may be necessary. Tooth #7 needs additional care and may require referral again, but this question is asking only about her bleeding problem in general.

2. **b**   A sufficient amount of plaque biofilm arouses suspicion that the bleeding is associated with plaque biofilm, but the possible effect of stress on Ms. Tevus should not be discounted. Option **a:** The reported symptoms do not include pain, ulceration, or a particularly descriptive aspect of the tissue, such as cratering. Option **c:** This case provided no description of linear gingival erythema, nor did the health history reveal any problem, such as human immunodeficiency virus infection, that might contribute to this choice. Option **d:** Her health history and age, the quantity of plaque biofilm, and the disposition of her gingivitis do not indicate a sex hormone influence.

3. **a**   Her plaque biofilm index is higher than acceptable. Option **b:** Nothing indicates that Ms. Tevus is not trying at home; indications are only that her efforts are not sufficiently effective to control bleeding. Option **c:** Her health history does not reflect an immunocompromised system. Option **d:** This reason may be subtle—but not obvious—for the reduced host resistance and the increased bleeding.

4. **b**   A mouthrinse such as essential oil or chlorhexidine digluconate (CHX) would be an option for this patient to assist her with mechanical plaque control. Option **a** is not a treatment for controlling plaque biofilm and gingivitis. It is an accepted adjunctive therapy for chronic periodontitis. Option **c** is not correct because she demonstrates acceptable technique with the toothbrush and interdental brush. Option **d** is beneficial for dental decay but is not indicated for the control of plaque biofilm and gingivitis.

5. **e**   An essential oil can be purchased over the counter and is economical to use initially. If the patient can use an alcohol mouthrinse and is not sensitive to the rinse, then essential oil has been shown to be effective and has ADA approval. However, CHX is also a good choice and is considered the gold standard for controlling plaque biofilm and gingivitis. It is a prescription rinse. Option **c** is not as effective as option **a** or **b.** Option **d** has no evidence for effectiveness.

6. **b**   A toothpaste with triclosan is easy to use and can be incorporated into the patient's home care with ease. The triclosan toothpaste has shown a substantial reduction in plaque biofilm and gingivitis and might be effective along with the anti–plaque biofilm mouthrinse. Option **a:** Because the patient has no evidence of root decay, an irrigant with a fluoride is probably not needed. Option **c:** Local delivery of antibiotics or antimicrobials is not warranted in this case because the bleeding is generalized throughout the mouth. Option **d** might be helpful for this patient but is not likely to resolve the bleeding problem.

7. **c**   This answer is preferred in the order listed. None of the other options are incorrect procedures; the

sequence of care is important. In reality, when the patient continued to exhibit bleeding and gingivitis problems, intervention with chemotherapeutics should have been considered earlier. Option **a:** Because irrigation has not been used, it might be used in this case. Debridement should always occur before other adjunctive therapies. In addition, debridement is necessary at this appointment because the patient may have a local irritant, such as calculus in the pocket. Because Ms. Tevus received professional debridement regularly, calculus with its accompanying plaque biofilm should not be the cause of the flare-up. In addition, the location and shape of the cingulum and lingual groove on this tooth, and on the tooth itself, should be reevaluated. Option **d:** If chemotherapeutics do not reverse the trend Ms. Tevus has experienced since surgery, then she should be referred back to the periodontist.

8. **a** Research with locally administered antibiotics or antimicrobials (LAAs) shows that they may need to be used more than one time to achieve clinically significant results. Each time an LAA product is used, the tooth should be thoroughly debrided and scaled and the root planed before placing the drug in the pocket. This procedure will ensure that the plaque biofilm has been removed thoroughly and then the drug can kill or suppress the remaining bacteria. The home care of the patient is essential to achieving a good result. Option **c** is also fine; however, with a 7-mm pocket, a second attempt with an LAA is acceptable. Option **c:** In this case, if the first three treatment options do not work, then the patient can then be referred to a specialist. Option **d:** An LAA should never be placed in a pocket without prior debridement or scaling. LAAs are considered adjunctive treatments and, as such, should be used after scaling, debridement, or both.

CHAPTER 28

1. **a** Mechanical bonding results when the resin sealant material becomes physically entrapped within the widened enamel pores. The application of a phosphoric acid solution removes inorganic materials and creates microporcs that increase the surface area of the enamel to form a strong bond between the resin and the enamel.

2. **d** Clinical research has shown sealants to be effective when adequately evaluated, maintained, and replaced. Research has also shown that early carious lesions can be safely arrested. Research regarding the use and effectiveness of sealants as a cost-effective preventive measure is overwhelming when compared with the cost and time required for operative treatment.

3. **c** Air-polishing used during a regular prophylaxis has been shown to increase the amount of wear on resin sealants. Air-polishing can create resin surface roughness, leading to future material breakdown. The amount of wear is increased with the time and exposure to air abrasion.

4. **a** A routine clinical evaluation is necessary to determine whether resealing of teeth is necessary in cases of sealant loss caused by poor retention. This issue is reflective of the sensitivity with the technique used to apply sealants to the surfaces of teeth. Any form or amount of moisture contamination can influence the overall effectiveness and resultant use of a sealant. Short-term sealant loss is often a result of technical application error rather than inadequate mechanical bonding. The inability to maintain a dry field is the most frequent reason sealants fail; poor isolation and improper acid-etching contribute to short-term loss.

5. **e** Inadequate enamel preparation increases the chances for marginal leakage and stains. Contamination of the field allows for marginal microleakage that leads to material breakdown and extrinsic stain trapping. Excessive material placement provides an area for the accumulation of plaque biofilm and stain. The stress from occlusion forced at the marginal sites allows the material to flex, which leads to marginal breakdown.

6. **a** If replacement of sealant materials becomes necessary as a result of inadequate bond strength or wear, any residual sealant material should be removed, if possible, and then the tooth should be cleansed, etched again, and treated by placing and curing new resin.

CHAPTER 29

1. **e** Nicotine mimics acetylcholine, which is a neurotransmitter that works throughout the body. Pharmacologic texts, nicotine-replacement pharmaceutical product materials, and other references describe this general action in more detail.

2. **c** Option **c** is a conservative statement in terms of the number of individuals exposed to nicotine who later develop dependence. More people who try nicotine become dependent —approximately one half— compared with lesser percentages among those who try other substances.

3. **d** Nicotine is a peripheral vasoconstrictor. Indeed, the absence of modest gingival bleeding often masks the development of serious periodontal problems.

4. **e** Almost daily, new evidence is reported about how smoking adversely affects the quality of life. In dentistry, all aspects of patient care are affected to a higher degree among smokers than among nonsmokers.

5. **b** Evidence presented in both the 1996 Agency for Health Care Policy and Research clinical practice guideline, *Smoking Cessation,* and the 2000 Public Health Service clinical practice guideline, *Treating Tobacco Use and Dependence,* makes it clear that the methods used—not the discipline of the user—are the key factor in effective treatment of people who attempt to stop tobacco use.

6. **c** The *attack* step is the exception. This chapter emphasized the use of a supportive approach, which requires the clinician to ask, assess, advise, assist, and arrange.

7. **d** Option **d** is the only answer that lists the U.S. Food and Drug Administration-approved methods presented in this chapter but is not meant to be all-inclusive. For example, the nasal

spray form of nicotine-replacement therapy is not mentioned.

8. **e** Most people require multiple attempts to quit. The experience of relapse actually increases the chance of achieving long-term abstinence.

9. **b** The most critical contact should occur shortly after the quit date when individuals reach their peak withdrawal symptoms. Recovery from acute conditions, such as from toxic gases, is measured in days. Some effects, such as cognitive and motor functions, may require weeks to recover. A few effects, such as craving precipitated by environmental cues, may remain throughout life.

10. **c** The American Dental Association does not associate with the tobacco industry.

CHAPTER 30

1. **d** Commercial denture cleansers contain powerful bleaching agents (sodium hypochlorite and sodium perborate) that leave a dull-gray deposit on the chrome-cobalt framework of partial dentures if the prostheses are left in the solution for more than 15 minutes a day.

2. **b** Many patients find the somewhat metallic aftertaste of stannous fluoride products, which is caused by tin ion, objectionable.

3. **b** Although the introduction of a fluoride product raises the fluoride concentration throughout the mouth, this patient should use the carrier on the mandibular arch because this area is the location of the teeth most susceptible to root caries, and these teeth need the most intense exposure to fluoride.

4. **b** Splint bars are often in direct contact with the adjacent oral mucosa, either because they were designed this way or because poor oral hygiene leads to edema. Unless the patient has been educated on using a floss threader or an interproximal cleansing brush, the surface of the bar adjacent to the soft tissue will probably harbor undisturbed plaque biofilm that irritates the mucosa.

5. **d** Saliva possesses antifungal and buffering properties; it is an effective lubricant. In a patient with a denture who has a dry mouth, candidal infection is likely to occur because the commensal pathogens are not inhibited from proliferating. The lower oral pH caused by the absence of acid buffers is favorable for candidal growth. The soft tissue, traumatized as the denture shifts against it, is prone to irritation by the metabolic by-products of the fungal colonies.

6. **d** The patient displays healthy gingival tissue despite his dry mouth; he clearly is effectively controlling plaque biofilm with his current regimen. His fixed bridgework likely necessitates using an interproximal cleaning aid or a floss threader anyway—and the more complex regimens are, the less likely they are to be followed than straightforward ones. The patient displays functional limitations (as a result of hand and shoulder arthritis) that impair his abilities to floss.

CHAPTER 31

1. **c** 4341 is the Current Dental Terminology code for scaling and root planing.

2. **c** The best time to evaluate the *current* status of self-care is before treatment because of disruption of bacterial accumulations in the treatment phase of therapy. Some evaluation will be an ongoing event occurring not only before treatment, but also during and after treatment and can be reviewed and discussed with the patient as needed throughout the appointment.

3. **a** Water is necessary in magnetostrictive units to cool the hand piece and the tip during instrumentation. Water also serves as an irrigant to lavage the working area during instrumentation.

4. **e** All of the items listed can be used to disrupt the bacterial biofilm to varying degrees of thoroughness and effectiveness.

5. **d** Nonadherent plaque biofilm is composed of both gram-positive and gram-negative species, which are virulent and can invade the periodontal tissues and secrete a large number of by-products that can damage host tissues, invoking an immune response that can cause further damage.

6. **a** Dental plaque biofilm and calculus are removed or managed in the treatment phase of periodontal debridement.

7. **d** The advanced lesion histologically exhibits extensive destruction of collagen fibers, predominance of plasma cell, regeneration of transseptal fibers as lesion moves apically and clinically as continued progression of gingivitis with attachment loss, and crestal alveolar bone resorbing.

8. **c** The healing rate of each structure is listed as follows:

Junctional epithelium	5 days
Sulcular epithelium	7-10 days
Gingival surface epithelium	**10-14 days**
Connective tissue	21-28 days
Bone	4-6 weeks

9. **e** Probing depth reduction is the only way (of the indicators listed) to determine clinically that an area has responded to treatment and is healing. Increased probing depth, gingival inflammation, and bleeding all indicate active disease. A high plaque biofilm index indicates neither healing nor disease but is never a good sign when healing is evaluated.

10. **c** Cavitation is a unique feature of water in powered instrumentation. Cavitation is a physiologic property associated with the operation of the ultrasonic generator causing water to atomize as it passes over the vibrations of the moving tip creating air cavities that collapse and explode. This cavitational action has been shown to cause cell disruption within the periodontal pocket, supporting the goals of periodontal debridement.

11. **c** Powered instrumentation will remove stain and can irritate the pulp if the tip is not adequately cooled with an accompanying irrigant, but these are

not positive effects. Option **b:** Removal of calculus is accomplished with powered instrumentation but the organization of bacterial colonies is not. Therefore option **c,** *the disruption of bacterial plaque biofilm and the removal of calculus,* are both positive effects of powered instrumentation.

12. **b** Option **b:** Standard, supragingival tips are designed to help remove heavier ledges of calculus and stain. Furcation involvement is generally subgingival with complex root anatomy that requires precise and accurate instrumentation and is best served with a fine tip that has good tactile capabilities or the curved tips that will allow better access to the anatomical features. Options **c** and **d** are better accomplished with a perio-design tip that can access posterior areas, as well as the varying anatomical features and debridement needs of the entire mouth.

13. **b** *Low-moderate power* is appropriate and acceptable for thinner insert tips, preferring the lowest power setting to accomplish the clinical needs of the case. High power is *never* recommended for thinner perio-type inserts or tips. Higher power can cause stresses within the metal of the thin tips and cause damage if not breakage.

14. **b** Administering a preprocedural rinse is recommended to reduce the level of bacteria in the aerosol generated during power instrumentation.

15. **c** If, during activation of the magnetostrictive instrument, the hand piece begins to feel warm, then some adjustment is required. Increasing the water flow may reduce the heat; however, disadvantages are that this produces too much water for the clinician and patient, and the spray will no longer be directed onto the tip. Reducing the power setting may also decrease the generation of heat to the hand piece but may result in inefficient deposit removal. Minor adjustments to water settings, power settings, or both can often manage the problem.

16. **b** Options **a, c,** and **d** all are associated with piezoelectric instruments. Option **b:** *Elliptical motion* is the only option that is associated with magnetostrictive technology.

17. **a** The power setting on the unit affects the length of stroke or amplitude of the vibrations. The higher power setting delivers a longer, more powerful stroke, and conversely, a lower power setting delivers a shorter, less powerful stroke. Because of the variation in tip size and clinical application, power settings need to be adjusted appropriately for each tip application on every powered scaling instrument.

CHAPTER 32

1. **d** All of the suggested polishing agents are indicated for Mr. Smith. An air-powder polisher is appropriate for stain removal on lingual and palatal surfaces with heavy stain. Coarse prophylaxis paste may also be used for these surfaces. Diamond polishing paste is indicated for polishing esthetic restorations on maxillary anterior facial surfaces.

2. **c** Anterior esthetic porcelain surfaces should be polished first with diamond polishing paste. This can then be followed by coarser paste for the remaining surfaces or the air-powder polisher. Esthetic restorations should always be polished first to reduce the possibility of coarse abrasives that remain in the rubber cup, which is likely to scratch the esthetic surface.

3. **a** Mr. Smith's stain classification is considered environmental exogenous because the stain is most likely attributed to his smoking. Developmental endogenous tetracycline stains are also present but have been cosmetically treated with facial porcelain veneers placed on teeth #6 to #11.

4. **c** Asthma and other respiratory illnesses are a contraindication for the use of air-powder polishing because of the amount of aerosols produced by the procedure. Diabetes, mitral valve prolapse, and chronic migraines are not included in the list of health concerns associated with air-polishing.

5. **a** Green stain is a stain acquired from chromogenic bacteria and gingival hemorrhage that forms on the external surface of the tooth near the gingival hemorrhage.

6. **d** Factors that determine the abrasiveness and polishing potential of an agent include particle size, shape, hardness, and concentration.

7. **b** Reduce the speed of the engine polisher and make sure plenty of paste is in the rubber cup. All other options listed actually increase the frictional heat on the tooth surface.

8. **c** Disadvantages of the Porte polisher are that the technique requires considerable hand strength and control and is a slow, tedious process.

9. **b** Polishing of unexposed root surfaces produces a therapeutic effect because the procedure is done to remove toxins from the unexposed root surfaces, which should result in a decrease in disease parameters.

CHAPTER 33

1. **d** The facial surfaces at the cervical region of the tooth are most sensitive to various forms of stimuli. This is caused by dentin exposure from gingival recession, abrasion, erosion, and abfraction, most of which are more prevalent on the facial surfaces and affect the cervical region of the tooth.

2. **c** Both statements are true. Many factors cause dentin hypersensitivity.

3. **a** Although interfering with the nerve fibers at the dentinal-pulpal junction is believed by some to be the mechanism of action of potassium nitrate, this is not the most accepted theory for the effectiveness of desensitizing agents. Occlusion of the dentinal tubules is the most accepted theory.

4. **b** Failure to determine the cause of dentinal hypersensitivity may result in recurrence or failure of treatment. Unfortunately, unlike management strategies for dental caries and periodontal disease, management strategies for dentinal hypersensitivity are not based on clinical data but on the logic derived from the cur-

rent understanding of the nature of the cause and risk factors for the condition.

5. **b** Burnishing is the process of creating a smear layer of dentin or other substances over and into the open dentinal tubules. Although burnishing alone can create some reduction in pain from hypersensitive dentin, the treatment is preferable and will last longer if an approved product for reduction of hypersensitivity is burnished into the dentin.

6. **c** Although all of the products listed have been shown to provide some reduction in dentin hypersensitivity, potassium nitrate seems to be longer lasting with less equivocal research findings.

CHAPTER 34

1. **d** Gut sutures are categorized as natural absorbable sutures and are digested by body enzymes and macrophages. In contrast, synthetic absorbable sutures are broken down by hydrolysis, a process during which water penetrates into the suture and contributes to its breakdown.

2. **c** Black silk sutures were used to adapt the free soft tissue graft closely to its underlying nutrient supply and to help stabilize the graft.

3. **b** Nonabsorbable silk sutures are commonly used in dentistry because of their exceptional handling characteristics that include flexibility, pliability, easy manipulation, and superior knot-holding capability.

4. **e** Although no one suture material is considered perfect for every dental need, the ideal suture material inhibits bacterial growth and adverse tissue reactions, maintains strength with decreasing size, is comfortable and easy to manipulate, can be sterilized and conveniently packaged, knots easily, is not adversely affected by products within the oral cavity, and is noncarcinogenic and nonallergenic.

5. **a** Literature has documented that eugenol-containing periodontal dressings contribute to delayed healing, inflammatory and allergic reactions, and tissue necrosis. Therefore modern periodontal dressings are usually formulated as noneugenol-containing products.

6. **d** The use and selection of a periodontal dressing is a personal choice of the dental healthcare provider. Ideal periodontal dressings set with dimensional stability allow easy manipulation, provide an acceptable taste, are nonirritating and nonallergenic, and discourage the accumulation of debris and bacteria.

7. **a** The continuous interlocking suture used in Case Study 34-1 incorporates both the facial and lingual flap into the suturing technique and the primary closure of the mesial and distal edentulous ridge adjacent to the remaining molar.

CHAPTER 35

1. **c** By definition, a Class II lesion and restoration is located on the proximal surface of a posterior tooth.

2. **c** The development of new dental materials has

afforded dental clinicians the opportunity to be much more conservative of natural tooth structure in the restorative process. Options **a, b,** and **d** are all results of this more conservative approach. Only option **c** is the result of a less conservative, *traditional* dental cavity preparation technique.

3. **a** By definition, amalgam is an alloy of mercury with any other metal. Silver (50% to 70%) and tin (15% to 30%) generally represent the largest percentage by weight of the remaining components in dental amalgam. Copper content varies widely, depending on whether the amalgam is a *low-copper* dental amalgam (2% to 5%) or a *high-copper* dental amalgam (12% to 30%).

4. **a** Resin composite was specifically designed to be a tooth-colored restorative material. Because this material is adhesively bonded to tooth structure, it generally results in lower microleakage than an amalgam restoration.

5. **b** The use of a wedge has no influence on the setting time of dental amalgam. The primary purpose of the wedge is to prevent amalgam from being over-packed beyond the gingival cavosurface margin that, if not confined to the preparation itself, would create an *overhang* of the metallic material. This would, in effect, create a plaque biofilm and bacteria trap that could initiate or perpetuate dental caries, periodontal disease, or both.

CHAPTER 36

1. **d** Composite resin systems can be used in the restoration of anterior or posterior teeth. They are best used in areas of small- to moderate-size defect, whether caused by decay, abrasion, erosion, or attrition factors.

2. **b** Anterior composite materials that have a high shine (e.g., mirofill, nanomers) can mimic enamel, are highly polishable, and leave the control and artistry of the restoration to the restoring dentist or hygienist.

3. **c** Acidulated phosphate fluoride has been shown to etch porcelain and may affect the filler particles in composite resins. Stannous fluoride may also cause discoloration of the restorations. Sodium fluoride treatments delivered after esthetic supportive care, after definitive restorative placement, and as part of self-care should be a component of all self-care education.

4. **d** A hygienist should consider the following guidelines when recommending or performing esthetic treatment options: Material selection must occur with the individual patient's specific situation and location in the mouth; the technique and modality used for tooth preparation; the restoration fabrication used; the luting and bonding agent used; and the restorative clinician's skill, judgment, and expertise.

5. **c** Most composite and ceramic materials reflect, refract, absorb, or transmit light rays differently from enamel and dentin; transillumination can be used to visually distinguish restorations. A simple technique to check margins can be achieved with the use of a

small surgical suction tip (preferably plastic), and the skill of detecting marginal discrepancies is greatly enhanced when the clinician uses magnification loupes.

6. **b** Protecting the definitive restoration and esthetic result may require fitting the patient for a protective night guard or traditional acrylic guard. Orthodontic treatment planning for an appliance should be incorporated into the restorative plan, before beginning the restorative or esthetic phase.

7. **a** Traditional prophylaxis pastes were never created for polishing esthetic restorations. Prophy paste may roughen, scratch, and dull the surface of tooth-colored restorative material. Acrylic material can be used during the provisional phase and is safe to be polished with prophy paste.

8. **b** Only the 10% carbamide peroxide solution has gained the American Dental Association (ADA) Seal of Acceptance. Several concentrations and materials have been clinically researched but have not sought ADA approval.

9. **b** The scalloped tray is trimmed following the contour of the tooth at the gingival-tooth interface. Therefore the solution is less likely to have direct contact with the gingival tissues.

10. **b** In-office professional bleaching uses a higher concentration of solution and heat to produce a fast "power" bleaching effect.

11. **d** Hydrogen peroxide (H_2O_2) is the correct answer. The other items are popular ingredients in bleaching gels but do not break down as H_2O_2.

12. **a** Whitening strips are convenient, easy to use, more economical, and better tolerated. An inherent disadvantage of whitening strips is that they cover only the facial surface of the anterior teeth.

13. **c** Poor substantivity or retention in bleaching trays occurred because of the fluidlike consistency of Proxigel. A more viscous gel-like material with better retention replaced Proxigel.

14. **d** Gingival irritation is the only consistent side effect of cosmetic whitening.

15. **d** Patient expectations should be realized *before* cosmetic whitening is begun. During treatment, the dental hygienist and dentist should be readily available for additional questions and concerns that might arise. After the procedure, the patient should be reminded that several factors determine how long the results will last, including consumption of chromogenic foods and tobacco use.

16. **d** Any of the options listed can help the sensitivity associated with tooth-bleaching procedures.

17. **b** The stain has been present since eruption, and the case information reveals that Jimmy has lived in a region typical of high levels of water fluoridation.

18. **a** A scalloped, reservoir tray can hold the bleaching agent on the area of Jimmy's tooth most in need of whitening.

19. **c** Third-degree tetracycline (TCN) stains are dark, gray-blue banding stains.

20. **a** A nonscalloped, nonreservoir tray design holds the bleaching agent against the gingival third of the tooth where the TCN stains are present on Ms. O'Bryan.

21. **c** Because cosmetic dental procedures should be completed after whitening procedures are complete, "composite on maxillary left incisor" is the most logical phase after bleaching therapy.

22. **b** Refer to the posttreatment intraoral photographs of Kathleen O'Bryan from Case Study 36-3.

23. **b** The use of professional strength whitening strips is a good recommendation for Ms. Randall, given her lack of personal free time and the area most noticeably yellow (six anterior teeth). Although tray bleaching is an option that might work for Ms. Randall, her busy schedule makes her a good candidate for the strip technology. A whitening dentifrice should be recommended for Ms. Randall, especially after the completion of a whitening procedure to help maintain her whiter smile. A whitening dentifrice, however, is not considered a tooth-whitening system. Although laser bleaching may be appropriate for Ms. Randall, the new professional-strength strip technology may be a better option for her because of convenience.

CHAPTER 37

1. **c** At 7 years of age, the patient should have his or her first permanent molars and incisors. At this time, an assessment is made of the relationship of the dentition and jaw. Before this time, these permanent teeth have not erupted and are not in occlusion. At the later time, the second permanent molars and other teeth have erupted. If space allocation is a problem, then determining this before having a full permanent dentition can make adjusting the situation easier or may involve less time to correct.

2. **e** All of the conditions listed would benefit from a two-phase approach. Each condition is complicated and requires significant change in either tooth location or bone growth. Thumb sucking can require an appliance and changing a habit.

3. **b** Facial mask therapy is used on individuals younger than age 21 years because the facial mask intervention is accomplished at an early age. Treatment effects are ultimately produced in the face and are incorporated into the future craniofacial growth that occurs over a long period.

4. **b** Orthognathic surgery is not something that is performed while the patient is in a mixed dentition—the maxilla and mandible are still growing. Until the skeletal growth is complete, surgery is not the option.

5. **c** Tooth bleaching or whitening on an orthodontic patient with fixed appliances would whiten only the portion of the tooth exposed, and the portion covered by the fixed appliance would be a different color when the appliance was removed.

6. **c** Although a maxillary diastema may be found in other races, it is more commonly found in blacks.

7. **d** A preorthodontic record is not expected to have

any of the diagnostic aids mentioned. However, once a patient has been selected for orthodontics, some of these diagnostic aids might be necessary to determine the appropriate treatment plan.

8. **c**   Root resorption during orthodontic tooth movement occurs when an unbalanced attack on the cementum of the root exists from appositional forces. Some root resorption occurs during movement but is not clinically evident. Severe root resorption, however, is rare; it occurs when forces are extreme or as a result of a genetic predisposition toward this problem. The more likely cause of severe *localized* root resorption occurs when maxillary incisors are forced against the lingual cortical plate.

9. **d**   Estimates from data obtained in the National Health and Nutritional Examination Survey (NHANES III) study suggest that, in the United States, more than one half of the population has some sort of malocclusion, which is based on the number of individuals receiving orthodontic treatment.

10. **d**   Angle's classification of occlusion identifies only the relationship between teeth and the occlusal plane relationship.

CHAPTER 38

1. **b**   The oral environment, including periodontal pockets, the posterior surface of the tongue, and the tonsil areas, harbors bacteria associated with 80% or more of chronic malodor. Halitosis refers to odor from the gastric tract; systemic causes of odor make up only 10% or less; and foods, medications, and so forth are considered extrinsic transitory causes.

2. **b**   Research has demonstrated that cleaning the tongue with a plastic scraper is not only more effective (removes greater amounts of biofilm from the tongue surface and oral cavity, eliminates translocation of biofilm from oral surfaces), but is also safer than using a toothbrush.

3. **c**   Volatile sulfer compounds (VSCs) are the odor-related gaseous by-products produced by gram-negative flora as it metabolizes proteins and amino acids.

4. **c**   Gram-negative bacteria are associated with periodontal infection because of their anaerobic nature and endotoxin and VSC production. Gram-positive aerobic flora is associated with both dental caries and gingivitis.

5. **b**   Gram-negative flora is responsible for VSC production, which increases with periodontal infections. Methyl mercaptan is produced at a higher concentration in persons with periodontal disease because of periodontal pocketing and an increased tongue coating.

6. **a**   VSC production is limited to flora from the coating on the tongue versus periodontal probing depths greater than 4 mm. Both hydrogen sulfide and methyl mercaptan are present, but in periodontally healthy mouths, additional hydrogen sulfide is produced.

7. **d**   VSCs not only produce detectable and offensive odor, but they are also involved in progression of infection and interfere with wound healing.

8. **c**   Zinc ions have a strong affinity for the thiol groups that are present in VSCs, which render them nonmalodorous by converting them to nonvolatile sulfides.

9. **a**   This buccal mucosa does not maintain an anaerobic environment for biofilm adherence versus subgingival spaces, crevices of the tongue, and the cryptic tissue of the tonsils.

10. **a**   In oral malodor prevention and treatment, optimal salivary flow is important. Therefore increasing salivary flow for persons who are experiencing oral malodor will be an important intervention and consideration.

CHAPTER 39

1. **e**   Prevention is not limited to preventing dental caries and periodontal disease. Primary care prevention should also include preventing traumatic dental injuries through the use of proper protective equipment and recognizing and reporting suspected child abuse and neglect.

2. **a**   Time is the most critical factor in successful reimplantation of avulsed teeth. This factor is directly related to maintaining the viability of the periodontal ligament cells.

3. **c**   Percussion only increases the traumatic insult to the already traumatized tooth and does not yield any useful diagnostic information.

4. **d**   Oral self-care is essential for the successful reattachment of tissue. The biofilm must be removed even though the tissues may be tender. This task is accomplished by using a soft toothbrush and is enhanced with an oral rinse.

5. **c**   Prevention is the key. An athlete is more likely to use a properly fitted mouthguard than one that is ill-fitting, causes gagging, inhibits speech, or obstructs breathing.

CHAPTER 40

1. **e**   All of these behaviors and conditions are characteristic of individuals who have dental fear. Fearful individuals are more likely than individuals without fear to cancel appointments on short notice, to appear indifferent, to avoid preventive care, and to display poor oral health status.

2. **c**   Assessing the patient's anxiety by using a valid and reliable dental anxiety inventory or questionnaire is the first step in treatment. Many questionnaires are formulated to ascertain a patient's level of anxiety and to determine a patient's anxiety-provoking stimuli. Questionnaires also identify which anxiety-reduction strategy to use.

3. **a**   Children between the ages of 3 and 5 years do not have the cognitive ability to understand detailed explanations or to engage in paced breathing. Coaxing is not recommended for children. Because children learn by

watching others, modeling is the most effective strategy for a mild-to-moderately anxious 3- to 5-year-old child. The most effective model is a peer of the same age.

4. **b** In systematic desensitization, a hierarchy of fear-producing situations related to the specific fear is generated. Starting with the least-feared stimulus, patients gradually progress through all items in the hierarchy while maintaining a relaxed state, which eventually enables them to cope effectively with the previously feared situation.

5. **c** The interpersonal relationship between the patient and the provider has the greatest effect on the patient's perceptions of the oral care experience. Once rapport and trust have been established, detailed information about the proposed treatment can assist with anxiety reduction and continued development of the patient-provider relationship.

CHAPTER 41

1. **d** The smaller the lumen is, the more pressure will be needed to establish a positive aspiration. The clinician might not use enough pressure with a 30-gauge needle to determine needle presence in a vessel adequately. Considering that aspiration is the most important safety step before deposing the anesthetic, a 25-gauge needle will give more reliable results than the other needles and increases safety in highly vascular areas.

2. **b** As the cell returns to its resting state, the membrane decreases permeability to sodium and potassium. The process of active transfer is needed to rebalance the extracellular and axoplasm fluids chemically and electronically. This mechanism is referred to as the *sodium pump*.

3. **d** Infected tissues have a lower pH, which limits the number of base molecules of anesthesia that are available to penetrate the nerve membrane. Because the passage of base molecules through the membrane is key to the success of nerve conduction blockade, limiting the number of base molecules limits the effectiveness of the anesthetic agent.

4. **e** Trismus is defined as a prolonged restricted opening of the mouth that may have a variety of causes. Postoperative inflammation or infection (or both) from dental procedures is among the causes and may result from irritation caused by excessive volumes of solutions injected into tissues, irritation resulting toxic chemical agents such as alcohol, irritation caused by pathogenic organisms on contaminated needles, and hematomas that can cause localized tissue irritation.

CHAPTER 42

1. **a** Nitrous oxide (N_2O) pressure in the tank will not show a decrease on the gauge until the liquid phase is nearly gone and primarily vapor remains in the tank.

2. **a** Tingling in the extremities is a symptom some patients experience during ideal sedation.

3. **d** Because N_2O is nonirritating to mucosa, it does not initiate asthmatic attacks.

4. **c** The reservoir bag expands and contracts concurrently with the patient's inhalations and exhalations.

5. **c** N_2O is almost completely eliminated via the lungs. No significant amount of the drug is metabolized in the body.

6. **d** When assessing recovery, the patient must feel normal. Continue to administer 100% oxygen until the patient reports "feeling fine." Postoperative vital signs also must be within close range of preoperative values.

7. **c** Following manufacturers' instructions regarding their specific equipment is always recommended; however, a general guideline of 2 years has been suggested for equipment evaluation.

8. **b** Recirculating ventilation systems only move the air to another area within the office and do not effectively remove the trace gas.

9. **a** N_2O is indicated for a hypersensitive gag reflex as discussed with Mr. Gruenwald in Case Study 42-1.

CHAPTER 43

1. **d** The many properties of saliva are listed in the introduction of this chapter. These properties include normal digesting, tasting, swallowing, speaking, and chewing.

2. **b** Saliva has numerous protective properties that include lubrication, antimicrobial activity, maintenance of pH and tooth integrity, debridement, maintenance of healthy mucous membranes, and maintenance of the oral flora.

3. **c** The parotid gland, the largest of the three glands, contributes approximately 25% of the total salivary secretions, is innervated by cranial nerve IX (glossopharyngeal nerve), and is serous in salivary secretions.

4. **c** Patients with decreased salivary gland function usually avoid eating spicy foods because the spicy foods exacerbate or increase the pain and burning of the tissues in the oral cavity.

5. **d** The patient with decreased salivary function has diminished protective activities from the saliva. Collectively, the end result can be an increased risk and rate of dental caries. To prevent this condition, the dental hygienist must (1) insist on meticulous oral hygiene from this patient, including the daily use of fluoride; (2) provide nutritional counseling to decrease the patient's carbohydrate intake; and (3) establish a frequent patient recall program, such as every 3 months or more frequently.

6. **a** Of the 200 most-prescribed medications in 1998, 55 list xerostomia as an expected adverse effect; 8 list the subjective complaint of glossodynia and glossitis; and another 15 list dysgeusia, or altered taste.

7. **a** The primary role of sialoperoxidase is to interfere with bacterial metabolism, and lysozyme attacks the cell wall of susceptible bacteria. Secretory immunoglobulin A (SIgA) targets specific bacterial antigens

275

and assists in blocking bacterial colonization. Histatins produce antimicrobial activity and may help neutralize enzymes of bacterial origin. Mucins provide lubrication and can cause bacteria to aggregate.

CHAPTER 44

1. **d** Using a mouth prop is simple, quick, and noninvasive and usually works. If not, then pursue further options.
2. **d** Taking the steps in options **a, b,** and **c** should minimize the development of new problems or the exacerbation of pressure points and reduce the possibility of decubitus ulcer formation.
3. **c** Air-polishing generates significant amounts of dry, powdered aerosols (generally sodium bicarbonate), which irritate the bronchi and may trigger a respiratory crisis.
4. **d** Either a kink in the line or a collection bag placed higher than the patient's bladder may impede urinary drainage. (This condition may also be exacerbated by the diuretic medication.) Option **b** is certainly permissible but generally not as appropriate as option **d.**
5. **a** If the patient frequently forgets basic personal care, another source should then be incorporated. Options **b, c,** and **d** are likely to be of little or no help.
6. **a** Radiographs are known to contribute to the formation of cataracts when the lens of the eye is directly exposed; therefore the operator should use caution (for both medical and legal reasons) when the patient is exposed to the x-rays. A well-collimated positioning indicating device and careful direction of the beam away from the lens is indicated. Air-polishing should be used only with adequate eye protection, as with any other patient.
7. **e** Options **a** and **c** are easy to try, and they maintain the patient's dignity. Pencils, notepads, and picture boards should only be offered after the initial attempts to communicate fail.
8. **e** Attention to these and other factors ensures compliance with the Americans with Disabilities Act regulations and facilitates the delivery of routine dental care to the broadest possible patient population.

CHAPTER 45

1. **c** Sertraline (Zoloft) is the only selective serotonin reuptake inhibitor (SSRI). Bupropion (Wellbutrin) and nefazodone (Serzone) are atypical. Phenelzine sulfate (Nardil) is a monoamine oxidase inhibitor; (MAOI); imipramine (Tofranil) is a tricyclic.
2. **c** Mysophobia is the fear of germs; *acrophobia* is the fear of heights; *claustrophobia* is the fear of confinement; *demophobia,* also known as *ochlophobia,* is the fear of crowds; *haphephobia* is the fear of being touched.
3. **d** Posttraumatic stress disorder (PTSD) occurs when a person experiences a negative life event beyond that individual's ability to cope.
4. **d** In bulimia nervosa the patient consumes large

quantities of food, followed by purging of that food in an effort to prevent weight gain.
5. **b** A hallucination is a perceptual experience in the absence of external stimulation, such as hearing voices that do not actually exist.
6. **a** The *Diagnostic and Statistical Manual of Mental Disorders,* fourth edition, text revision *(DSM-IV-TR)* is the manual developed by the American Psychiatric Association (APA) that names and categorizes more than 200 mental disorders.
7. **c** Antipsychotic medications have been shown to cause tardive dyskinesia (TD) in approximately 25% of patients within 3 months of treatment initiation.
8. **c** A sense of entitlement is one of the diagnostic criteria for narcissistic personality disorder, not for a major depressive episode.

CHAPTER 46

1. **d** Sjögren's syndrome (SS) is characterized by the triad of xerostomia, keratoconjunctivitis sicca (KCS), and a connective tissue disorder.
2. **b** Individuals with SS have a higher incidence of hypothyroidism.
3. **c** Studies of patients with SS have demonstrated significantly higher plaque biofilm index scores and dental caries rates and increased alveolar bone loss. However, whether these increased risks are the result of hyposalivation or the presence of autoimmune disease is unclear.
4. **c** Rheumatoid arthritis (RA) is characterized by synovitis, erosion of bone, joint deformity, and loss of joint mobility.
5. **a** Temporomandibular joint (TMJ) involvement is the most common oral sign of RA.
6. **b** The malar "butterfly" rash is the classic sign of systemic lupus erythematosus (SLE).
7. **c** Patients with SLE should be treated with caution, especially if they have renal or cardiovascular complications. Prophylactic antibiotics may be indicated if the patient has low white blood cell (WBC) counts, is taking immunosuppressive medications, or has valve abnormalities.
8. **a** Patients with autoimmune disease are often treated with supplemental steroid therapy, which requires a booster dose during oral health care to prevent adrenal crisis.
9. **d** Limited scleroderma tends to be a feature of CREST syndrome.
10. **a** Microstomia may cause a limitation of the opening of the mandible by 70%, making oral hygiene care challenging for both the patient and the clinician.
11. **d** Individuals with type 1 diabetes mellitus (DM) produce no endogenous insulin; therefore they are insulin dependent.
12. **b** Patients with type 1 DM who are treated during the peak activity period of insulin therapy are at risk of a hypoglycemic emergency.
13. **c** Thyrotoxic crisis or thyroid storm is the greatest

concern when treating patients with hyperthryroidism. Untreated or poorly controlled patients are susceptible to this medical emergency.

14. **b**   Both hyperthyroidism and hypothyroidism may produce a goiter. Surgery is not the treatment of choice for either condition.

15. **c**   Myasthenia gravis (MG) causes profound weakness of the muscles of mastication.

CHAPTER 47

1. **c**   Human immunodeficiency virus (HIV) is a retrovirus and uses ribonucleic acid (RNA) to replicate.

2. **d**   All of the choices are characteristic of HIV infection.

3. **d**   The other conditions are not fungal infections. The most common fungal infection associated with HIV is oropharyngeal candidiasis.

4. **c**   During the highly active antiretroviral therapy (HAART) era, oral warts increased and are caused by the human papillomavirus.

5. **a**   Labial and buccal mucosa, ventral surface of the tongue, posterior oropharynx, and maxillary and mandibular vestibules are the locations for aphthous ulcers. All of these tissues are nonfixed or nonkeratinized tissues.

6. **b**   Sweat, unlike saliva, tears, and blood, has not been identified as an infectious body fluid and therefore does not require the use of standard precautions.

7. **c**   Biofilm found in dental unit waterlines is filled with many microorganisms that have been classified as opportunistic. Some of these organisms are pathogenic, and those with suppressed immune systems can become sick with respiratory or other infections from high-speed dental handpieces and powered scaling instruments.

8. **d**   Using all these methods is most effective to control biofilm in dental waterlines.

9. **d**   The Centers for Disease Control and Prevention (CDC) requires the use of sterile irrigants during surgical procedures.

10. **b**   The hepatitis vaccine became widely available in the 1980s and became a childhood vaccine in the 1990s.

11. **a**   Unvaccinated (susceptible) healthcare personnel who are exposed to rubella are restricted from the seventh day after the first exposure through the twenty-first day following the last exposure to the virus. This period is the time during which the exposed person might be infectious after exposure.

12. **c**   Unvaccinated (susceptible) healthcare personnel exposed to mumps are restricted from the twelfth day following the first exposure through the twenty-sixth day after the last exposure. This period is the time during which the exposed person could be infectious after exposure.

13. **e**   The Rehabilitation Act was passed in 1973, but HIV was not an issue at that time. In 1990, the Americans with Disabilities Act was passed, clarifying HIV as a handicapping condition.

14. **False**   Referral cannot be based on a provider's comfort level for treating a patient with HIV. Referral decisions must be based on the dental needs such as referrals to specialists in which the treatment needs can be delivered.

15 **True**   Universal precautions are not a modification to patient care but are standard operating procedure.

CHAPTER 48

1. **c**   Oral mucosal cells have a life span of 10 to 14 days. Radiation terminates the growth and replication of cancer cells by destroying the cell nucleus. Normal cells may also be affected, thereby dying at a faster rate than they are produced.

2. **c**   The mandible is more susceptible to osteoradionecrosis because it is denser and less vascular than the maxilla and consequently absorbs more radiation. Patients undergoing radiation doses in excess of 7000 cGy are at greater risk also. As in the case presented, the greatest risk is the patient whose mandible has received extensive radiation and requires tooth extractions after completing radiation therapy.

3. **b**   Because of the patient's prior exposure to radiation, hyperbaric oxygen treatments were scheduled to flood the tissues with oxygen and increase the blood supply, particularly to the extraction sites to decrease the risk of osteoradionecrosis.

4. **a**   1.23% acidulated phosphate fluoride is a relatively high concentration of fluoride that is recommended for application only once every 6 months.

5. **b**   A $T_2 N_0 M_0$ tumor is classified as stage II because the neoplasm has increased in size, but it has no lymph node involvement and no metastasis.

6. **d**   The brain, muscles, and spinal cord are the least affected by radiation. Cells of the bone marrow and alimentary tract divide rapidly and are easily destroyed by radiation.

7. **a**   Approximately 40% of patients receiving chemotherapy experience oral complications. Ulcerative mucositis is a common oral condition, particularly when the chemotherapy is aggressive, the drugs are stomatotoxic, and prolonged myelosuppression results.

8. **c**   The patient has a thrombocyte count of 18,000/mm^3. Spontaneous bleeding occurs at a platelet count of approximately 20,000/mm^3.

9. **a**   For dental treatment to occur safely, the neutrophil count must be at least 1000/mm^3. The existence of an indwelling catheter is an indication for antibiotic premedication.

10. **c**   Dental treatment procedures should be postponed unless the platelet count is at least 50,000/mm^3. Toothbrushing should involve the use of a supersoft nylon brush or gauze or cotton swabs dipped in warm water or 0.12% chlorhexidine gluconate when the platelet count drops below 20,000/mm^3.

11. **d**   Irradiation or prolonged intensive chemotherapy of the developing body, dentition, and facial bones may result in hypocalcification, enamel hypoplasia, delayed or arrested tooth development, premature

277

closure of root apices, microdontia, complete or partial anodontia, micrognathia, retrognathia, and skeletal and dental malocclusion.

CHAPTER 49

1. **c**   The 4355 (full-mouth debridement) insurance code should be used only if the patient has no periodontal attachment loss or the dental hygienist and dentist cannot complete a comprehensive oral evaluation because of the presence of heavy deposits.
2. **a**   You should use an intraoral camera to photograph restorative needs and areas of periodontal inflammation to engage the patient in the examination process. Engaging the patient in the examination process is educational and encourages the patient to become responsible for his or her own health.
3. **d**   The dental hygienist can enhance the patient's perceived value of dental hygiene services by involving the patient in the examination process by calling out the periodontal probe readings, by providing the patient with an oral hygiene fitness report (OHFR) at the conclusion of each supportive care visit, and by showing interest in the patient by remembering personal information such as family and work issues. All of these things create a patient-oriented practice, which is a prerequisite to a successful dental hygiene department.
4. **c**   Individualized treatment plans catering to each patient's specific needs are characteristic of a highly effective dental hygiene department. Patient recommendations and treatment should be based on correct diagnosis and treatment planning according to each individual's needs (as opposed to a "one-size-fits-all" approach). Furthermore, understanding a patient's concerns and fears will help the clinician determine what is best for the patient.
5. **b**   Mechanical polishing would be the best procedure to eliminate without compromising the patient's health or quality of the supportive care appointment (SCA). With the established links between periodontal inflammation and many systemic diseases, vital signs, oral cancer screenings, and complete periodontal examinations are integral parts of the SCA. In addition, they are good risk management practices. Mechanical polishing offers no health benefit to the patient, and current research mandates only selective polishing.

CHAPTER 50

1. **b**   Having polished, well-kept fingernails is not inappropriate for an interview. Long fingernails and *black* polish would not be appropriate, however. The other items are totally inappropriate.
2. **e**   All of the items are possible with an advanced degree.
3. **c**   Values are the foundation on which all other components of behavior are built.
4. **e**   The dental hygienist is not only a direct care provider, but also a disease-prevention and health-promotion specialist. He or she may also be an efficient healthcare provider, but this is not the best choice.
5. **b**   The professional portfolio may contain all the other components listed, but the intent is that of documentation to evaluate continued competence.
6. **c**   The greatest feeling a dental hygienist can have and the best thing a dental hygienist can do for patients is to educate them as to the association between oral and systemic diseases. This information empowers others to prevent disease and to promote wellness among even more people.

CHAPTER 51

1. **d**   Although all of the other choices have made impacts on either dentistry or dental hygiene, technological advances will have the greatest impact on future dental hygiene practice.
2. **b**   The association between systemic and oral diseases is important to health care but will be applied in dental, medical, and public health settings.
3. **c**   Leaders are needed with all of the listed characteristics, but these leaders should not work alone. Vision and implementation of ideas require more than just a leader to accomplish.
4. **a**   Both statements are true as the future of the dental hygienist is projected.
5. **b**   Although all of the characteristics in each option are appropriate for a leader to possess, affecting change is almost impossible without insight and commitment.
6. **d**   The National Dental Hygiene Research Agenda is both a list of research priorities as outlined by the ADHA and important to the progression of the dental hygiene profession.